YOGA FOR HEALTH AND RELAXATION

Published by:
Lotus Press Publishers & Distributors

YOGA FOR HEALTH AND RELAXATION

KRISHAN KUMAR SUMAN
Yogacharya, Ayurvedratna
Editor of Yogamanjari

Lotus PRESS
4735/22, Prakash Deep Building,
Ansari Road, Daryaganj,
New Delhi - 110002

Lotus Press Publishers & Distributors
Unit No 220, Second Floor,
4735/22, Prakash Deep Building,
Ansari Road, Darya Ganj, New Delhi-110002
Ph.: 23280047, 32903912, 098118-38000
E-mail: lotuspress1984@gmail.com
Visit us : www.lotuspress.co.in

YOGA FOR HEALTH AND RELAXATION

ISBN: 978-81-8382-322-7

Published by: **Lotus Press Publishers & Distributors,** New Delhi
Printed at: **Bharat Offset Works,** Delhi

Preface

Health is our birth right. It is said, 'prevention is better than cure'. Health can't be maintained by taking pills. Health can't be purchased. Yoga is the best way to achieve a good health.

There are 16 chapter in this book—'Yoga for Health and Relaxation'. The fundamental knowledge is given in this book. All the necessary matter is given for health and relaxation.

- 'What is Yoga' is described according 'Yoga Sutra' and 'Bhagwad Gita', Swami Vivekanand and Swami Vishnu-Devananda, Swami Yogananda and Swami Satyananda Saraswati were the ambassadors of yoga to bring it in America and other countries.
- **Branches of Yoga:** There are many branches are working in different styles as—Astanga yoga, Iyengar, Yoga, Viniyoga, Anusarayoga (based on attitude, allignment and action), Ananda yoga, Bikram yoga, Integral yoga, Jivamukti, Kali Ray Triyoga, Shivananda Yoga, Kripalu, Swaroopa and Kundalini yoga are described in brief.
- **Types of Yoga:** There are 8 types of yoga are described in this chapter as—Jnana, Karma, Bhakti, Laya, Raja, Mantra, Tantra and Hatha Yoga in brief.

- **The Eight limbs of yoga:** Patanjali's eightfold path of yoga offers guidelines for a meaningful and purpose ful life. These eight limbs are Yama, Niyama, Asana, Parnayama, Pratyahara, Dharana, Dhyana and Samadhi (8 types) are explained in brief.
- **Five Principles of Yoga:** Five main principles are base of yogabhyasa as—Proper relaxation, proper exercise, proper breathing, proper diet (yogic Ahara), positive thinking and meditation.
- **Benefits of Yoga** are explained in a clear way. The benefits of Yoga are numerous, including physical fitness, stress control, general well being mental clarity and greater self understanding, About 25 benefits are given in this chapter. Ten psychological benefits and 10 biochemical benefits are told. Yoga and exercise comparision is also given in 12 points.
- **Stretching exercises** for health and beauty are very helful. 7 yogasanas are given for the fitness of the neck, arms, legs, chest and waist to unwind all the stiff muscles.
- **Asanas** bring physical as well as mental stability health and vigour. Asanas basically, perform five foundations like conative, cognitive, mental, intellectual and spiritual. Eight catagories of asanas are listed. 39 yogasanas are explained with figures.
- **Surya Namaskar** is the famous and traditional exercise of 12 postures. It limbers up the whole body in preparation for the yogasanas. Twelve figures are given with mantras.
- **Pranayama** is explained in sub headings assesntial knowledge (place, time, posture and bath), benefits

of pranayama, techniques of pranayamas, 3 bandhas, process of pranayama and 12 prayanamas are explained with method. Panchpranas also listed.

- **Meditation** is the need of the day. 4 Mantras are told for meditation to chant for preparation. It removes the stress and provides relaxation.
- **Weight regulation** is the need of the child, men and women. Seven yogasanas are recommended pranayama too is very beneficial in weight reducing.
- **Yoga diet:** Yoga is the only Science that has laid great emphasis on food. Yoga and Ayurveda advise on sattvic food which is vegetarian. Yoga food have been classified as rajsic, tamsic and sattvic. Food to eat (ten points), foods to avoid, fasting are discussed clearly.
- **Yoga for all** is necessary for men, women, yoga for elderly and yoga for children are explained. For men 13 yogasanas and Ujjayi breathing are recommended. For women 18 yogasanas and Kapalbhati pranayama are suggested for elderly persons, four yogasanas and kapalbhati pranayama are told useful, like this children also can perform Shirshasana, dancer's pose and Kandharasana for.good health.
- **Mental health** is peace of mind. What is mental health, more positive approaches (6 points), 19 characteristics of sound mental health, causes and symptoms of mental ill health, healing needs, 13 Negative habits and attitude should be changed into positive habits, rules for a sound mental health are discussed fairly. 21 points are given to be mentally healthy.

- **The art of relaxation** is an important skill in yoga. Some relaxing techniques are given in this chapter. Relaxing yogasanas, breathing exercises for relaxation of heart and mind are described efficiently.

This book is a good guide to every learner of yoga. The reader who practise those yogic techniques can get good health, mental peace and happiness.

❑❑❑

Table of Contents

Other Books on

HEALTH BOOKS

1. Child Development (New)	195/-
2. Yoga For Daily Life (New)	295/-
3. A Guide to Your Pregnancy (New)	175/-
4. Ayurveda for All (New)	175/-
5. A Guide to Migraine, Airthritis, Cervical Spondylosis, and Backache (New)	125/-
6. Body and Beauty Care (New)	125/-
7. Yoga for All (New)	250/-
8. Child Care and Nutrition	125/-
9. Naturopathy Modern Way of Life	125/-
10. First Aid How to Handle an Accident	125/-
11. Acupressure in Daily Life	125/-
12. Complete Book of Yoga	150/-
13. Look Younger at Any Age	125/-
14. HIV/AIDS - Transmission, Prevention & Alternative Therapies	110/-
15. Diabetics and Diet	110/-
16. Increase your Height & Loose your Weight	125/-
17. Make Fitness A Way of Life	195/-
18. Common Problems of Children	160/-
19. Handbook of Nutrition & Dietetics	250/-
20. A Guide to Massage Therapy	125/-
21. A Guide to Family Medicine	150/-
22. A Guide to Digestive Disorders	125/-
23. Complete Book of Child Care	150/-
24. A Guide to Homoeopathy	125/-
25. Life Begins at 40	125/-
26. Alternative Therapies	125/-
27. How to Overcome Stress	125/-
28. Yoga Therapy	225/-
29. Obesity	125/-
30. Self Motivation	125/-
31. Yoga for Health and Relaxation	160/-
32. Women Disorders and Pregnancy	125/-
33. A Guide to Body Pains	125/-
34. Sex Education	125/-
35. Common Diseases and Cure	125/-
36. Pranayama for Better Life	125/-
37. Herbal Home Remedies	125/-
38. A Guide to Beauty & Skin Care	125/-
39. A Guide to Heart Care	125/-
40. A Guide to High Blood Pressure	125/-
41. Cancer Causes and Prevention	125/-
42. Nature Cure for Common Diseases	125/-
43. Good Health Through Food and Regimen	110/-
44. A Guide to Allergies	125/-
45. A Guide to Aging	125/-
46. Ayurveda for Health & Beauty	125/-

1

WHAT IS YOGA?

The word 'yoga', from the Sanskrit word *yuj*, means to yoke or bind, and is often interpreted as 'union' or a method of discipline. A male who practises yoga is called a yogi, and a female practitioner, a yogini. The Indian sage Patanjali is believed to have collated the practice of yoga into the *Yoga Sutra* nearly 2,000 years ago. The *Sutra* is a collection of 295 statements that serves as a philosophical guidebook for most of the yoga that is practised today.

Yoga is not a religion. The *Yoga Sutra* provides a framework for spatial growth and mastery over the physical and mental body. Yoga sometimes interweaves other philosophies such as Hinduism or Buddhism. It is not necessary to surrender your own religious beliefs to practise yoga.

In the *Bhagavad Gita,* which is the most important authority on yoga philosophy, Lord Krishna explains to Arjuna the meaning of yoga as a deliverance from contact with pain and sorrow.

When the restlessness of the mind, intellect and self is stilled through the practice of yoga, the yogi, by the grace of the spirit within himself, finds fulfilment. When the senses are stilled, when the mind is at rest, when the intellect wavers not, then is reached the highest state. Yoga has also been described as wisdom in work or skilful living among activities with harmony and moderation. All the ancient commentaries on yoga have stressed that it is essential to work under the direction of a guru (teacher, master).

Swami Vishnu-Devananda says, "The yogi regards the physical body as an instrument for his journey toward perfection." Yoga is a science of health. The teachings of yoga are based on intricate and precise understanding of the healthy functioning of the human body and mind. Its techniques are designed to maximise your potential for good health, vitality and lasting youthfulness.

The history of yoga is long and steeped in tradition. Contrary to what some people may believe, yoga was not developed as the newest way to slim down so they could fit into smaller-size pants. Yoga originated in India, and the first mention of it is made in the *Riġ Veda*, one of the sacred texts of Hinduism.

Swami Vivekananda added to the history of yoga by taking it to America, when he addressed the Parliament of World Religions in 1893, and discussed the path of yoga. As a result of his speech, it quickly began to blossom as a practice in many areas of the country. Yoga has since gained major popularily in the United States and other Western countries.

Today, the focus is more on yoga's practical benefits. There is a definite difference between yoga and stretching and normal exercises. Traditional exercises are oriented towards a certain goal, such as doing a number of sit-ups or push-ups; yoga, on the other hand, is a process. It teaches the concept of focusing your awareness while performing specific postures or asanas.

Many people think that they need to be flexible to begin yoga, but that's a little bit like thinking that you need to be able to play tennis in order to take tennis lessons. All you really need to begin practising yoga is your body, mind, and a bit of curiosity.

Today, the most popular form of yoga is a Hathayoga which refers to the metaphysical and physical aspects of yoga. Our physical and mental facilities must be so trained that they function with rhythm and harmony. 'Ha' and 'Tha' mean the moon and the sun respectively. The perfection of health is the first condition but the radiant health is of a greater or higher order, for the objective is always super-physical, including the soul or spirit and every psychic manifestation associated with the functioning of the nervous system. The popularity of the Hathayoga is due to its insistence on health.

Yoga classes consist mostly of the practice of traditional physical exercises or asanas. Breathing practices are also essential for better health, and form an integral part of the practice. A class often includes some meditation, with relaxation as the final sequence.

Yoga, however, does not just adhere to the pursuit of metaphysics, but goes beyond it, transcending the ego in order to awaken the spirit within, the pure being of consciousness and awareness. It is the exercise of discipline, the practice of purification, wherein the yogi aspires to transcend the ego into the pure self, balance, consciousness, centring its deepest awareness to the point of liberation. It is the path to happiness, health and tranquillity.

❑❑❑

2

BRANCHES OF YOGA

Yoga varies greatly depending on what is emphasized. Some forms focus on strict body alignment, others on holding postures. Many approaches highlight the importance of the flow from one posture to another, and how the execution of each pose coordinates with the movement of the breath (this is called *Vinyasa* and can be used with any yoga form).

Yoga continues to evolve through the years to meet the needs of every individual from self-realisation to curing of various ailments. Through the years, Hathayoga, which is the most popular form of yoga worldwide, continues to evolve and flourish. It is the branch of yoga that focuses on the physical well-being of a person and believes that the body is the vehicle of the spirit. A lot of different yoga styles rooted from Hathayoga. All these styles aim to balance the mind, the body and the spirit through the asanas or poses; however, the emphasis varies. Some put emphases on the strict alignment of the body while some focus on the coordination of breath and movement.

All these yoga styles have common roots. In fact, the founder of the major styles—Ashtanga, Iyengar and Viniyoga—were all students of Krishnamachary, a famous teacher of the Yoga Institute at the Mysore Palace in India.

The other styles, like Integral and Sivananda, were created by disciples of the famous guru Sivananda. No style is better than another.

As you consider the possibilities and methods of yoga, bear your own nature in mind. Remember, yoga is designed to enable you to begin from your immediate present state of consciousness, and move forward day by day, into a state of wholeness, well-being and enlightenment. Even the beginner is able to overcome physical or mental tension, and progress towards a life of higher consciousness. An integral yoga ensures that your body, mind and soul are in perfect harmony. Realise fitness, freedom from stress and happiness, all through yoga, in the years to come.

There are various branches of yoga which are given in detail below.

Anusara

The word 'Anusara' means 'flowing with grace'; it also means 'to step into the current Divine Will', 'following your heart', or 'to move with the current of Divine Will'. This new form of yoga, developed by John Friend, is both physically demanding and spiritually fulfilling. It is believed to be grounded in deep knowledge of outer and inner alignment. It is a combination of Hathayoga and biochemical principles; in other words, it is an integrated approach to Hathayoga in which the human spirit blends with the precise science of biochemics. It can be therapeutically effective and physically transformative. The central philosophy of this yoga is that each person is equally divine in every part of body, mind and spirit. Each student's various abilities and limitations are respected and honoured. In practising this yoga, you must keep your heart open, and flow with grace as you do the postures. Anusara focuses on pose that bind muscular strength and stability. The student is encouraged to perform them with an integrated awareness of all parts of the body.

Anusara yoga practice is based on three principles: attitude, alignment and action, making it different from Hathayoga.

Attitude: The student of yoga balances an opening to grace with an aspiration for awakening to his true nature.

Alignment: Each pose is performed with an integrated awareness of all the different parts of the body.

Action: Each pose is performed with an artistic expression of the heart in which muscular stability is balanced with an expansive inner freedom.

Ananda

For those who strive for higher goals than merely maintaining physical fitness, Ananda Yoga provides a tool for spiritual growth while releasing unwanted tensions. Swami Kriyananda developed this particular style of yoga during the 1960's after returning to California following a period of intense yoga training under Guru Paramahansa Yogananda. The most unique part of this system is the use of silent affirmations while holding a pose. The affirmations are intended to help deepen and enhance the subtle benefits of each asana, providing a technique for aligning body, energy and mind. The instructors guide their students through a series of gentle Hatha postures, designed to move energy upward to the brain, preparing the body for meditation. The focus is also on proper alignment, easeful posture transitions, and pranayama (controlled breathing exercises), to facilitate an exploration into the inner dimensions of yoga and self-awareness.

Ashtanga

The term 'Ashtanga' comes from the *Yoga Sutra* of Patanjali, where it refers to classical yoga's eight (*ashta*) limb (*anga*) practice. Some yoga scholars, like George Feuerstein, maintain that Patanjali's real contribution to yoga was Kriya Yoga, the 'yoga of internal action' and the eight-limb practice was borrowed from another source. The eight limbs are restraint, observance, posture, breath, control, sense withdrawal, concentration, meditative absorption and 'ecstasy', meaning 'standing inside of'. This last word is Mircea Eliade's translation of *samadhi*, which literally means to 'put together' or 'bring into harmony'. In *samadhi*, we 'stand inside of' our true Self in preparation for the ultimate state of classical yoga, the eternal 'aloneness' (*kaivalya*) of the Self in the purity and joy of its being.

While Patanjali's underlying dualism between self and nature has long been out of favour, his eight-limb method still influences many modern schools of yoga. One of those schools in the currently popular Ashtanga Yoga developed by K. Pattabhi Jois from the techniques of T. Krishnacharya. It is modelled on the eight-limb practice of Patanjali. The emphasis, however, is on the correct performance of the third limb (posture) as a means of realising all the limbs, including, of course *samadhi*. Pattabhi calls his system 'Ashtanga' in part to encourage his students to look into the whole practice more deeply, and integrate all the limbs.

Ashtanga Yoga is physically demanding. The student moves through a series of flows, jumping from one posture to another in order to build strength, flexibility and stamina. It is not for beginners or anyone who has been taking a leisurely approach to fitness. It involves performing a challenging sequence of poses with Ujjayi breathing in *vinyasa* (a flow of postures).

The system is based on six series of asanas which increase in difficulty, allowing students to work at their own pace. This will help them achieve increased strength, flexibility and stamina. The so-called power yoga is based on Ashtanga.

Bikram

Bikram Yoga is named after its founder, Bikram Choudhary. It is a series of 26 poses performed in a room heated to around 100° F, aptly dubbed as 'hot yoga'. The sauna-like atmosphere is intended to warm up the muscles, so that they are easier to stretch without injury. This yoga is considered to be an all-round workout that builds cardiovascular fitness as well as muscular strength and endurance.

Each yoga pose is usually performed twice and held for a certain duration of time. The yoga sessions start from standing postures, then the back bends, forward bends and twists. The poses are in tune with Kapalabhati Breath or the 'breath of five'.

Heat is used in this yoga to allow you to go deeper and safer into a yoga pose. Your body becomes more flexible in the hot room, and eliminates the risk for injuries, while promoting the release of toxins from your body, and flexibility. Yoga also works on your internal organs like the glands and the nervous system.

Bikram Yoga is designed to scientifically warm and stretch muscular ligaments and tendons in the order in which they should be stretched. It also helps in reducing stress and increasing blood circulation, as well as losing weight, and developing toned and strong muscles. Bikram

Yoga is not about being flexible, but about strengthening your body and your spine in all directions with the goal of creating a union between the body, mind and spirit.

Integral

Integral Yoga focuses on pranayama (breath control), meditation and asanas (physical poses). This style of yoga was developed by Swami Sacchidananda in 1966. He introduced to an entire generation of young people his yogic philosophy: "an easeful body, a peaceful mind and a useful life". His goal was to help people integrate yoga's teachings into their everyday work and relationships, which he hoped would promote greater peace and tolerance worldwide.

Integral Yoga uses classical Hatha postures, which are meant to be performed as a meditation, balancing physical effort and relaxation. It is also used for therapeutical purposes.

The practice of Integral Yoga evolves around eight main goals, which are:

1. Physical health and strength
2. Control over all senses
3. Clear, calm and well-disciplined mind
4. Higher level of intellect
5. Strong and pliable will
6. Love and compassion
7. Purer ego
8. Ultimate peace and joy

Iyengar

Iyengar Yoga is named after B.K.S. Iyengar who is one of the best-known yoga teachers, and who is also the creator of the most popular styles of yoga in the world.

Iyengar's style is noted for great attention to detail and precise alignment of postures. Poses here are generally held longer than any other forms of yoga, and repeated several times. The 80-year-old yoga master encourages his students to penetrate deeper into the experience of each pose. This is the trademark of Iyengar Yoga—an intense focus on the subtle of each posture. The students can pay close attention to the precise muscular and skeletal alignment this system demands.

Also specific to this system of yoga is the use of props, including belts, chains, blocks and blankets, to help accommodate any special needs such as injuries or structural imbalances. In forward bends, for example, if someone's hamstrings aren't flexible, he or she can use a prop to help extend the spine. The wall is often used for support in a variety of poses.

Only when one achieves a certain level of mastery of these poses can one move to pranayama. One of the most popular poses in Iyengar Yoga is the 'Tadasana or the Mountain pose.'

Jivamukti

This yoga method was created by David Life and Sharon Gannon in 1984. It is a vigorously physical and intellectually stimulating yoga leading to spiritual awareness. It combines an Ashtanga background with a variety of ancient and modern spiritual techniques. In addition to Vinyasa-style asanas, classes include chanting, meditation, readings, music and affirmations. There are also specialised courses in Sanskrit and the sacred yoga texts.

Beginner classes start by emphasizing standing poses, followed by instruction on forward bends, back bends and inversions, these classes also introduce chants.

Kali Ray Triyoga

A series of flowing, dance-like movements intuitively came to Kali Ray while leading group meditation in 1980. In 1986, after developing these movements into seven distinct levels, he established the Triyoga Centre in California, offering a system of yoga that is taught in a meditative environment.

The first level is a slow, relaxing and rejuvenating practice. The class, often accompanied by music, focuses on natural alignment and breath within the flow, and ends with meditation. A union of asana, pranayama and *mudra* (seals), this practice is deeply meditative, promoting relaxation and inner peace. The exercises combine flowing and sustained postures following a spinal wave-like movement, economy of motion, and synchronised breath and mudra. Students may progress from basic to advance as they increase their flexibility, strength, endurance and knowledge of the flows.

Kripalu

Located in the Berkshire region of western Massachusetts, the Kripalu Centre for Yoga and Health has guided thousands of people along their path of self-discovery by teaching a system of yoga developed over a 20-year period by yogi Amrit Desai and the Kripalu staff.

Kripalu Yoga is also called the yoga of consciousness Kripalu puts great emphasis on proper breath, alignment, coordination of breath and movement, and 'honouring the wisdom of the body'—you work according to the limits of your individual flexibility and strength. Alignment follows awareness. Students learn to focus on the physical and psychological reactions caused by various postures to develop their awareness of mind, body, emotion and spirit.

There are three stages in Kripalu Yoga. Stage one is wilful practice whereby you learn the postures, proper breathing and explore your body's abilities. Stage two is wilful surrender involving holding the postures for an extended time, developing concentration and awareness of your thoughts and emotions. The final stage is meditation in motion in which the movement from one posture to another arises unconsciously and spontaneously while you are in a meditative state.

Kundalini Yoga

Kundalini Yoga, stemming from the Tantra Yoga path, at one time remained a closely-guarded secret practised by a select few. In 1969, however, yogi Bhajan decided to change this tradition by bringing Kundalini to the West. His reasoning was based on the philosophy that it's everybody's birthright to be 'healthy, happy and holy', and he believed Kundalini would help spiritual seekers from all religious paths to tap into their great potential.

The practice of Kundalini Yoga incorporates postures, dynamic breathing techniques, and chanting and meditating on mantras, such as 'Sat Nam' (meaning 'I am truth'). Practitioners concentrate on awakening the energy at the base of the spine, and drawing it upward through each of the seven chakras.

In this form of yoga, sequences of fast movements are done for fairly long periods of time. Repetition and speed make Kundalini extremely aerobic.

The emphasis however is not on the yoga poses, but on the chanting and breathing. Kundalini Yoga rewards yogis with spiritual transformation and unity consciousness.

Sivananda

At its core, Sivananda Yoga is geared towards helping students answer the age-old questions "Who am I?" This yoga practice is based on the philosophy of Swami Sivananda of Rishikesh, India, who taught disciples to "serve, love, give, purify, meditate, realise." In order to achieve this goal, he advocated a path that would recognise and synthesise each level of the human experience, including the intellect, heart, body and mind.

In 1957, his disciple, Vishnu-Devananda introduced these teachings to an American audience, and founded the International Sivananda Yoga Vedanta Centers, summarising Sivananda's system into five main principles:

1. Proper exercises (asanas)
2. Proper breathing (pranayama)
3. Proper relaxation (shavasana)
4. Proper diet (vegetarian)
5. Positive thinking (vedanta) and meditation (dhyana).

There are more than 80 centres worldwide as well as ashrams and teacher-training programms, all of which follow a Hathayoga practice consisting of 12 basic yoga poses that seek to increase strength, flexibility, proper breathing and meditation. Chanting pranayama and meditation help the students to release stress and blocked energy.

Svaroopa

This yoga was developed by Rama Berch, who founded and directs the Master Yoga Academy, and created the yoga programme for Dr. Deepak Chopra's Center for Well Being, both located in La Jolla, California.

Svaroopa Yoga teaches significantly different ways of doing familiar poses, emphasizing the opening of the spine by beginning at the tailbone and progressing through each spinal area in turn. Every pose incorporates principles of asana, anatomy and yoga philosophy. It also emphasizes the development of transcendent inner experience, which is called Svaroopa by Patanjali in the *Yoga Sutra*. This is a consciousness-oriented yoga that also promotes healing and transformation. Svaroopa yoga is not an athletic endeavour, but a development of consciousness using the body as a tool.

Viniyoga

Viniyoga, or what is also known as the 'yoga for wellness', rooted from the principle practised by T. Krishnamachari, that is, to develop practices for individual conditions and purposes. His son, T.K.V. Desikachar, continued this principle, and developed the practice of Viniyoga.

Viniyoga is an empowering and transformative practice designed to help address and integrate the transitions at all levels—physically, emotionally and intellectually. It is a methodology for developing an integrated practice for each person's needs as they grow and change. As children, our practice should support balanced growth and development of the body and mind; as adults, it should protect our health and promote our ability to be productive in the world. And as seniors, it should help us maintain health and inspire a deeper quest for self-realisation.

Viniyoga makes use of modified yoga poses that are designed to meet the specific needs of an individual, and to enhance healing, flexibility and strength of joints. Viniyoga poses also intend to promote the feeling of well-being and strength. Practices may include pranayama, meditation, reflection, study and other classic elements, but the emphasis is on coordination of breath and movement.

❑❑❑

3

TYPES OF YOGA

Whether you are devotional or intellectual in nature, yoga has a path for you. In ancient times, yoga was often referred to a tree, a living entity with roots, a trunk, branches, blossoms and fruit. The branches are jnana yoga, karma yoga, raja yoga, mantra yoga, tantra yoga, laya yoga, hathayoga and bhakti yoga. The other less important yogas are sankhya (yoga of science of numbers), sanyasa (yoga of renunciation), dhyana (yoga of meditation), vijnas (yoga of comprehension), abhyasa (yoga of study effort), budhi (yoga of wisdom), and atman (yoga of self).

Each branch has its unique characteristics and function, representing a particular approach to life. Some people may find one particular branch more inviting than another. However, it is important to note that involvement in one of these paths does not preclude activity in any of the others, and in fact you will find many paths regularly overlapping.

Jnana Yoga

Jnana Yoga is the path of spiritual knowledge, selflessness and strength coming from faith and experience in the oneness of all.

Jnana Yoga is closely related to raja yoga. It is regarded to be metaphysical, and the most difficult of the paths of yoga. A higher level of consciousness can help you to resolve the intellectual mysteries, paradoxes and contradictions that you comfront in life. What is needed to tread this path smoothly are purity of thought, concentration and meditation. You need to lead a detached life, without getting entangled in emotions, stresses and cares of the world. You have to delve behind the illusory veil that hides the truth. In Jnana Yoga you can find answers to metaphysical queries.

When a thought or feeling occurs that is not relevant to your meditative goal, you have to keep discarding it time and again patiently until the mind is clear and the soul is revealed.

Karma Yoga

Karma Yoga is the path of action, work, activity, and enterprise. 'Karma' means action which includes action and reaction. It is a path on which tread the worker, mechanic, inventor, doctor, businessman, teacher, farmer, and so on. It is the yoga of action inspired with an ideal. It lays emphasis on adoption of righteous means to achieve righteous ends. Good actions motivated by good intentions must be carried out without the expectation of results or rewards.

Karma Yoga focuses on harnessing of cumulative energy. Just as water leaking or dripping from taps goes to waste, similarly actions that encourage negative energies, like jealousy, anger, greed, etc., can cause frittering away of energy.

Karma Yoga is the path of service, and none of us can escape this pathway. The principle of Karma Yoga is that what we experience today is created by our actions in the past. Being aware of this, all of our present efforts become a way to consciously create a future that frees us from being bound by negativity and selfishness. Karma is the path of self-transcending action. We practise Karma Yoga whenever we perform our work and live our lives in a selfless fashion, and as a way to serve others.

Raja Yoga

'Raja' means 'royal', and meditation is the focal point of this branch of yoga. This approach involves strict adherence to the eight 'limbs' of yoga as outlined by Patanjali in the *Yoga Sutras*.

Raja Yoga attracts individuals who are introspective and drawn to meditation. Members of religious orders and spiritual communities devote themselves to this branch of yoga. However, even though this path suggests a monastic or contemplative lifestyle, entering an ashram or monastery is not a prerequisite to practising Raja Yoga.

Mantra Yoga

Mantra Yoga in the science of sounds and vibrations. It involves chanting and incantation, the repetition of sacred mantras, and the effects of them on one's mind and emotions.

The most popular among the mantras is 'Om'. Om is a mantra of vibration, that is traditionally chanted at the beginning and end of yoga sessions. It is said to be the sound of the universe.

Everything that exists pulsates, creating a rhythmic vibration that the ancient yogis acknowledged with the sound of Om. We may not always be aware of this sound in our daily lives, but we can hear it in the rustling of the autumn leaves, the waves on the shore, the inside of a seashell.

Chanting 'Om' allows us to recognise our experience as a reflection of how the whole universe moves—the setting sun, the rising moon, the ebb and flow of the tides, the beating of our hearts. As we chant 'Om', it takes us for a ride on this universal movement, through our breath, our awareness and our physical energy, and we begin to sense a bigger connection that is both uplifting and soothing.

Laya Yoga

Laya Yoga is the study of energy in the human organism and the mystery of the life force, inclusive of bodily heat and sexual powers. All of us have energy centres in a body, called *chakras*. These chakras function like windows or doorways that lead to higher levels of consciousness.

When your heart chakra, for example, opens up through meditation, you experience an awareness of love flowing out, overcoming selfishness and self-centredness. The energy emanating from it gives you tremendous strength and insight to transcend fears and worries. Similarly, the energy from the other chakras equips you to deal with the mundane and rise to a higher consciousness.

Tantra Yoga

Tantra Yoga is the yoga of designs and symbols. The word 'tantra' means 'expansion'. A yogi practising this yoga focuses on expanding all levels of his or her consciousness to realise the supreme reality. Tantra deals with the dynamic aspect of divinity called *shakti*, or the 'Cosmic Mother'.

The tantric yogi strives to release all the negative blocks that are latent in him by attuning himself with the spiritual dynamic energy. He seeks the creative force and transmutes this energy into higher channels.

Hathayoga

Hathayoga is an ideal system for attaining harmonious development of body, mind and soul—perfect physical and mental health this involves concentration breath control, endurance, flexibility and stretching, aligning and strengthening the mind and awakening the spirit. The word 'Hatha' means wilful or forceful. It refers to a set of physical exercises or postures, and sequence of asanas designed to align your skin, muscles and bones. The postures are also designed to open many channels of the body—especially the main channel, the spine—so that energy can flow freely.

Hatha is also translated as 'ha' meaning 'sun' and 'tha' meaning 'moon'. This refers to the balance of the masculine aspects (active, hot, sun) and feminine aspects (receptive, cool, moon) within all of us. Hathayoga is a path toward creating balance and uniting opposites. In our physical bodies we develop a balance of strength and flexibility. We also learn to balance our effort, and surrender in each pose.

Hathayoga is a powerful tool for self-transformation. It asks us to bring our attention to our breath, which helps us to still the fluctuations of the mind, and be more present in the unfolding of each moment.

Bhakti Yoga

Bhakti Yoga is the approach to God through worship, adoration and self-abnegation. It is the most natural path for those who are seeking emotional fulfilment and well-being. It is the path taken by visionaries, mystic poets, saints and sufis of all religions.

Bhakti Yoga is based on the philosophy of love. Swami Vivekananda described it as 'real, genuine search after the Lord, a search beginning, continuing and ending in love'. One of the principles of Bhakti Yoga is to 'love all and hate none'. It requires a renunciation of all worldly things and attachments. Love of God and all his creatures is the main focus of this yoga.

❑❑❑

4

THE EIGHT LIMBS OF YOGA

Patanjali's eightfold path of yoga offers guidelines for a meaningful and purposeful life. In his *Yoga Sutra*, the eightfold path is called Ashtanga, which literally means 'eight limbs' (*ashta* = eight, *anga* = limb). These eight steps basically act as guidelines on how to live a meaningful and purposeful life. They serve as a prescription for moral and ethical conduct and self-discipline. They direct attention towards one's health, and they help us to acknowledge the spiritual aspects of our nature.

The eight limbs are yama, niyama, asana, pranayama, pratyahara, dharana, dhyana and samadhi.

Yama

Yama means restraint or abstention, and deals with universal moral commandments, with one's ethical stands and sense of integrity, focusing on one's behaviour and how one conducts oneself in life. One should abstain from such vices as vices, stealing, greed, lust and so on.

Patanjali, the father of yoga, states that the harmonious development of body, mind and soul can be obtained through the eight limbs of yoga, and stresses on moral conduct, truthfulness and non-covetousness that are essential ingredients to reach a higher level of consciousness.

Yamas are universal practices that relate best to what we know as the golden rule: "Do unto others as you would have them do unto you." The five yamas are:

1. **Ahimsa:** Non-violence, meaning not to hurt any creature mentally or physically through mind, speech or action.
2. **Satya:** Truthfulness, the presentation of matter as perceived with the help of sense organs.
3. **Asteya:** Non-stealing, meaning not to covet and acquire physically, mentally or by speech, others' possessions.
4. **Bramacharya:** Continence, or moderation in sex between married couples.
5. **Aparigraha:** Non-acquisitiveness, meaning abandoning wealth and means of sensual pleasure.

Niyama

Niyama, the second limb, has to do with self-discipline and spiritual observances. Regularly attending temple or church services, developing your own personal meditation practices, or making a habit of taking contemplative walks are all examples of niyamas in practice. This leads to developing devotion, purity, studiousness, contentment and discipline.

There are five niyamas, which are as follows:

1. **Saucha**: Cleanliness, meaning internal and external purification of the body and the mind.
2. **Santosha**: Contentment, meaning a state of mind by which one lives happily and satisfied in congenial or uncongenial atmosphere.
3. **Tapas**: Austerity or penance which is the conquest of all desires or sensual pleasures by practising purity in thought, speech and action.

4. **Avadhyaya**: Study of the sacred scriptures and of one's self. It means exchange of thoughts in order to secure purity in thought and accomplish knowledge.
5. **Ishwara Pranidhana**: Surrender to God, meaning having pure devotion to God, and surrendering all actions to him.

Asana

Asanas, the postures practised in yoga, comprise the third limb. In the yogic view, the body is the temple of spirit, the care of which is an important stage of our spiritual growth. Through the practice of asanas, we develop the habit of discipline and the ability to concentrate, both of which are necessary for meditation.

Pranayama

Generally translated as breath control, this fourth limb consists of techniques designed to gain mastery over the respiratory process while recognising the connection between the breath, the mind and the emotions. As implied by the literal translation of pranayama—life force extension—yogis believe that it not only rejuvenates the body but also actually extends life itself. You can practise pranayama as an isolated technique, that is, simply sitting and performing a number of breathing exercises, or integrate it into your daily Hathayoga routine.

Pratyahara

This means sense withdrawal, or turning the senses inward and withdrawing them from external objects. It is a discipline of the senses, whereby the extroversion of the sense organs due to their hankering after worldly objects has to be restrained. It is essential to practise pratyahara for achieving the three meditative stages of dharma, dhyana and samadhi. Perfecting this technique of yoga is also essential in order to break out from the eternal cycle of rebirths.

Dharana

Dharana is concentration, or fixing the mind on one object at a place or point. In other words, you have to focus the pure mind on your personal deity or on the individual self. The practice of dharana helps the mind to focus and concentrate on a particular object.

The last three limbs of Ashtanga Yoga are the three essential stages of meditation. Dharana involves developing and extending our powers of concentration. This consists of various ways of directing and controlling our attention and mind-fixing skills, such as concentration on the chakras or turning inwards.

Dhyana

Dhyana, meaning meditation, saves the mind from dissipation, and takes it to the realm of peace and perfection. It awakens the slumbering energies of the mind. As you continue to meditate, the mind becomes pure; the old *samskaras* are dissolved; and the mind becomes free from impurities. You then progress from the unconscious to the subconscious state; from the subconscious to the superconscious state, that is, the state of *samadhi*.

Samadhi

Samadhi means merging with the universal consciousness. Samadhi, or total absorption, is the ability to become one with the true self, and merge into the object of concentration. In this state of mind, the perceiver and the other object of perception unite through the very act of perception—a true unity of all thought and action. This is the acme of all yogic endeavours—the ultimate yoga or connection between the individual and the universal soul. Patanjali's *Yoga Sutra* categorises and grades the levels of samadhi in the first chapter:

1. *Samprajnata samadhi,* or distinguished contemplation.
2. *Asamprajnata samadhi,* or non-distinguished contemplation.
3. *Savitarka samadhi,* or deliberated absorption.
4. *Nirvitarka samadhi,* or non-deliberated absorption.
5. *Savichara samadhi,* or reflective meditation.
6. *Nirvichara samadhi,* or non-reflective meditation.
7. *Sabija samadhi,* where the mind continues to carry seeds of earthly impressions.
8. *Nirbija samadhi,* where each seed of earthly impressions has been erased.

❑❑❑

5

FIVE PRINCIPLES OF YOGA

Yoga is one of the world's oldest branches of spiritual inquiry which is gaining popularity worldwide. Today, yoga classes are in high demand at health and fitness clubs, and in many spas. People are now very interested in mind-body forms of exercise. They are tired of pounding their bodies with exercise. And as the baby boomers get older, they are trying to soften their workouts a little, trying to balance themselves. Yoga fits in perfectly with that.

The five principles of yoga are the basis of attaining a healthy body and mind through the practice of yoga. Given below are the five principles of yoga.

1. Proper Relaxation

By releasing the tension in the muscles, and putting the whole body at rest, you revitalise your nervous system and achieve inner peace, making you feel relaxed and refreshed. This relaxed feeling is carried over into all your activities, and helps you conserve your energy, and let go of all worries and fears.

2. Proper Exercise

This principle revolves around the idea that our physical

body is meant to move and exercise. Proper exercise is achieved through the yoga posture or asana which systematically works on all parts of the body-structure and tones the muscles and ligaments, enhances the flexibility of the spine and the joints, and improves blood circulation. The asanas are designed to regulate the physical and physiological functions of the body.

Practising these yoga poses makes your body relaxed, gives you more strength and energy, and rejuvenates the various systems of the body.

The yoga posture goes together with proper breathing. Each movement and stretch should be guided by your breathe, making your movement and your breath coordinated and feel like one and the same. The execution of the asana is beneficial to the body, and at the same time, contributes to spiritual and mental growth.

3. Proper Breathing

This means breathing fully and rhythmically, making use of all the parts of your lungs to increase your oxygen intake. Proper breathing should be deep, slow and rhythmical. To achieve this, you need to be able to regulate the length and duration of our inhalation, exhalation and the retention of air in your lungs, or the pauses between breaths.

Yoga breathing exercise or pranayama teaches you how you can recharge your body and control your mental state by regulating the flow of prana the life force. This helps you achieve a calmer and more focused mind, and increases your energy level.

4. Proper Diet

What you eat extremely affects your mind. Improper diet results in mental inefficiency and blocks spiritual awareness. Proper diet is one that nourishes both mind and body. It should be well balanced and based on natural foods. Proper diet in yoga also means eating in moderation and eating only when you are hungry. We sometimes tend to eat when we are upset, using food to fill the gap or the emptiness that we feel. Bad eating habits will cause our senses to be so dull that we won't notice how much we eat or how it tastes, and may result in diet-related aliments like obesity and diabetes.

Food should keep the body light and supple, the mind calm, and it should also help in keeping a strong immune system.

5. Positive Thinking and Meditation

The way we think highly affects our way of life. Practise keeping a positive outlook in life, for this will facilitate in having a peaceful mind. Positive thinking and meditation help you remove negative thoughts, and put your mind under perfect control.

❑❑❑

6

BENEFITS OF YOGA

As studies continue to reveal yoga's many health benefits, this centuries-old eastern philosophy is fast becoming the new fitness soul-mate for workout enthusiasts. Contemporary devotees range from high-powered executives trying to keep hearts beating on a healthy note to image-conscious cine stars striving for sleek physiques. Even prominent athletes are adding yoga to their training regime to develop balanced, injury-free muscles and spines.

Yet to applaud yoga for its physical benefits alone would only diminish what this entire system has to offer as a whole. By practising yoga on a regular basis, you may be surprised to find that you are building much more than a strong, flexible body.

Most people are usually drawn to yoga first as a way to keep fit, but the idea behind the physical practice of yoga is to encourage deeper mind-body awareness. Healing and balancing the physical body helps bring clarity and focus to the mind as well.

Initially, the sole purpose of practising yoga was to experience spiritual enlightenment. In Sanskrit, yoga translates as 'yoke' or 'union', describing the integration of mind and body to create a greater connection with one's own pure, essential nature.

Yoga poses have been developed over centuries of research and experience. They have been found to be extremely effective in increasing flexibility of the body, and freeing all the energy blocks. Besides this, it leads to a healthier body. Helping to lose excess flab and weight is another great benefit. Massaging the internal organs of the body and the rarely stimulated parts, such as the thyroid gland, is beneficial. It also helps to treat severe health disorders—from common ones such as backaches and arthiritis to 'seemingly' unrelated disorders such as stammering.

It is recommended to include some form of yoga positions and preferably a yoga routine in your life. Meditation, pranayama, relaxation and cleansing are very important aspects of yoga, yet the most ignored. A complete yoga should include these aspects which result in huge benefits in terms of correcting metabolic disorders, overcoming stress and mind behaviours that seem beyond your control.

The benefits of yoga are numerous, including physical fitness, stress control, general well-being, mental clarity, and greater self-understanding. People of all ages can do yoga, and it can also be adapted for people with disabilities or special needs. The poses enhance muscle strength, coordination, flexibility and agility, and can help a bad back feel better. But that's not all. Regular practice of yoga helps to keep our body fit, controls cholesterol level, reduces weight, normalises blood pressure, and improves heart performance.

When people actively seek to reduce the stress in their lives by quieting the mind, the body often works to heal itself. In this sense, yoga can be seen not only as a way to get into shape on several levels, but also as a tool for self-healing. Other studies show that patients with heart problems who followed a stress-reduction programme that includes yoga did better than patients who exercised or did nothing. Further, preliminary studies in the US and India suggest that yoga may be helpful for specific conditions, such as asthma, epilepsy, anxiety, stress and others.

As for athletes, yoga can be a powerful enhancement in regular training exercises. Adding yoga in a routine training programme helps develop strength, flexibility, range of motion, concentration, cardiovascular health, and reduces stress, tension and tightness. The most significant benefit of adding yoga to a training programme is its effect on performance. Yoga allows an athlete to train harder and at a higher level because the range of motion is greater, and the fear of injury lessened.

The modern mantra regarding yoga and fitness is: increased overall health, energy and vitality; greater body awareness, a stronger and leaner body, increased flexibility with improved range of motion, better posture, natural weight loss, reduced stress and tension, improved concentration.

When using meditation for healing, it is a matter of resting your mind, clearing of all thought, and then using focus and breathing techniques to shut out all stresses and mundane thoughts of everyday life, with repeated effort, the goal of clearing your mind, to think of nothing, does occur and the process of meditation takes on its own energy. The result is peace, severity, calmness, and eventually opening yourself to new insights.

Yoga is aimed to unite the mind, body and spirit. Yogis is view that the mind and body are one, and that, if given the right tools and taken to the right environment, it can find harmony and heal itself. Yoga, therefore, is considered therapeutic. It helps you become more aware of your body's posture, alignment and patterns of movement. It makes the body more flexible, and helps you relax even in the midst of a stess-stricken environment. This is one of the foremost reasons why people want to start practising yoga—to feel fitter, be more energetic, and be happier and peaceful.

Yoga is a science that has been practised for thousands of years. It consists of ancient theories, observations and principles about the mind and body connection which is now being proven by modern medicine. Substantial research has been conducted to look at the health benefits of yoga—from the yoga postures (Asanas), yoga breathing (Pranayama) and meditation (Dhyana). The information is grouped into three categories: physiological, psychological, and biochemical effects.

Physiological Benefits

1. Yoga stabilises the autonomic nervous system equilibrium.
2. The pulse rate and respiratory rate decrease.
3. Laboratory tests have proved the yogi's increased abilities of consciously controlling autonomic or involuntary functions, such as blood pressure,

heartbeat and temperature. Some Asanas are designed to normalize your blood pressure.

The relaxation and exercise components of yoga have a major role to play in the treatment and prevention of hypertension. A combination of biofeedback and yogic breathing and relaxation techniques has been found to lower blood pressure, and reduce the need for high blood pressure medication in people suffering from it.

4. The galvanic skin response increases. Yoga gives your skin a healthy glow by balancing your hormones and boosting the flow of oxygen-rich blood to your skin. This keeps your skin resilient, and prevents dryness and excessive sagging. Yoga also tones the muscles of your face and neck.
5. Cardiovascular efficiency increases. Some yoga asanas are essential in the prevention of heart ailments. Backward-bending postures elevate the heart rate.
6. Respiratory efficiency increases. Patients who practise yoga have better chance of gaining the ability to control their breathing problems with the help of yogic breathing exercises. It is possible to control an attack of severe shortness of breath without having to seek medical help. Various studies have confirmed the beneficial effects of yoga for patients with respiratory problems.
7. Gastro-intestinal function normalises.
8. The endocrine function normalises.
9. The excretory functions improve.
10. Musculoskeletal flexibility and joint range of motion increase. Many people wonder if yoga can

improve their muscle fitness. They recognise that yoga can help reduce stress and increase flexibility, but when it comes to increasing muscles fitness, they think it might be a little too 'weak' to do the job. The fact is that yoga can definitely make you stronger.

Unlike traditional weight-building exercises, in yoga your body provides the resistance. While you are not likely to produce the build-up muscle of some weightlifters, you will certainly increase your muscle strength.

Many poses in yoga are done very slowly, or you stay in the posture for several breaths. It is much more challenging to your muscles to hold a pose, or do it slowly than it is to allow momentum to move you through an action. In addition, some balance postures require enormous muscle control in order to prevent you from falling over. This helps to build and strengthen your muscles.

Compared to weight training, the muscles you develop during yoga are more likely to be elongated, because, while you are strengthening them, you are simultaneously lengthening them. You also do not focus on an isolated muscle, but actively recruit the smaller muscle groups as well. You truly work your entire body when you practise yoga.

Practising yoga can help realign your muscles, so they are more balanced. Since you are not overworking any specific muscle group, you are less likely to get injured. In addition to all its other benefits, yoga can help you improve muscle fitness.

Whether you choose to use it as your primary means of strength training or you want it to supplement your other exercises, yoga can help your muscles grow fit, balanced and strong.

11. Yoga helps in breath-holding time. The breathing technique can make you feel refreshed, and cleanses the air passages which can help prevent respiratory ailments.
12. Joint range of motion increases.
13. Grip strength increases.
14. Eye-hand coordination improves, leading to a person's general well-being.
15. Dexterity, skills, reaction time and posture improve.
16. Strength, resilience and endurance increase.
17. Energy level and immunity increase.
18. Weight normalises, as it is possible to burn fat.
19. Sleep, sturdiness, balance, depth perception, and integrated functions of body parts improve.
20. Arthritis conditions and pain decrease.
21. Twisting postures stimulate the adrenal glands and flush out toxins.
22. Studies conducted at yoga institutions in India have reported impressive success in improving asthma. Physicians have found that the addition of improved concentration abilities and yogic meditation together with the practice of simple postures and pranayama make treatment more effective.
23. Yoga is believed to reduce pain by helping the brain's pain centre regulate the gate-controlling

mechanism located in the spinal cord and the secretion of natural pain-killers in the body. Breathing exercises used in yoga can also reduce pain. Since muscles tend to relax when you exhale, lengthening the time of exhalation can help produce relaxation and reduce tension. Awareness of breathing helps to achieve calmer, slower reputation, and aids in relaxation and pain management.

24. Back pain is the most common reason to seek medical attention. Yoga has consistently been used to cure and prevent back pain by enhancing strength and flexibility. Both acute and long-term stress can lead to muscle tension and exacerbate back problems.
25. Yoga's gentle exercise, designed to provide relief to needed joints, has been yoga's show-motion movements and gentle pressures reach deep into troubled joints. In addition, the easy stretches, in conjunction with deep breathing exercises, relieve the tension that binds up the muscles and further tightens the joints. Yoga is exercise and relaxation into one—the perfect anti-rheumatism and anti-arthritis formula.

Psychological Benefits

1. Somatic and kinesthetic awareness increase.
2. Mood improves and subjective well-being increases. Mental health and physical energy are difficult to quantify, but virtually everyone who participates in yoga over a period of time reports a positive effect on outlook and energy level. Yogic stretching and breathing exercises have been seen

to result in an invigorating effect on both mental and physical energy and improved mood. When you achieve the yogic spirit, you can begin knowing yourself to be at peace.

3. Self-acceptance and self-actualisation increase.
4. Social adjustment increases.
5. Anxiety and depression decrease, as also hostility towards others.
6. Concentration, memory and attention improve.
7. Self-awareness increases on both a physical and psychological level.
8. Communication skills and mental performance improve. A common technique used in yoga is breathing through one nostril at a time. EEG studies of the electrical impulses of the brain have shown that breathing through one nostril results in increased activity on the opposite side of the brain. Some experts suggest that the regular practice of breathing through one nostril may help improve communication between the right and left side of the brain. Studies have also shown that this increased brain activity is associated with better performance.
9. Learning efficiency, symbol coding, depth perception improve.
10. Yogic theory and practice lead to increased self-knowledge. This knowledge is not nearly that of the practical kind relating to techniques, but especially of a spiritual sort pertaining of grasping something about the nature of the self at rest.

Biochemical Benefits

1. Glucose level decreases.

2. The sodium level too decreases.
3. The total cholesterol decreases.
4. Triglycerides decrease.
5. HDL (high-density lipids) increases, while LDL (low-density lipids) decreases and VLDL (very low-density lipid) cholesterol decreases.
6. Cholinesterase increases.
7. Catecholamines decrease.
8. AT Pase, hemastocrit, haemoglobin and lymphocyte count increase.
9. Total white blood cell count decreases.
10. Thyroxin, vitamin C and total serum protein increase.

Yoga Benefits in Comparison to Exercise Benefits

Yoga	Exercise
1. Parasympathetic nervous system dominates.	1. Sympathetic nervous system dominates.
2. Subcortical regions of brain dominate.	2. Cortical regions of brain dominate.
3. Slow dynamic and static movement.	3. Rapid forceful movements.
4. Normalisation of muscle tone.	4. Increased muscle tension.
5. Low risk of injuring muscles and ligaments.	5. Higher risk of injury.
6. Low caloric consumption.	6. Moderate to high caloric consumption.
7. Effort minimised, relaxed.	7. Effort is maximised.
8. Energising (breathing is natural or controlled).	8. Fatiguing (breathing is taxed).

9. Balanced activity of opposing muscle groups.	9. Imbalanced activity of opposing groups.
10. Non-competitive, process oriented.	10. Competitive, goal-oriented.
11. Awareness is internal (focus is on breath and the infinite).	11. Awareness is external (focus is on reaching the toes, reaching the toes, reaching the finishing line, etc.).
12. Limitless possibilities for growth in self-awareness.	12. Boredom factor.

Yoga exercises not only free a great amount of tied up energy but bad emotional and mental relaxation. Once you start doing these exercises, you will begin to truly appreciate the inestimable value of yoga for promoting physical and mental fitness.

It is well to remember that most physical problems have developed over a period of time, months or years, and when attempting to deal with them through natural means, such as yoga, it is unrealistic to expect an immediate solution. If the laws of nature have been abused for prolonged periods, no sudden reversal of the resultant condition can be anticipated. It is possible that minor conditions will respond quickly; more serious problems require sustained, patient practice. However, you can be assured that in stimulating the lifeforce, you are increasing your organism's healing power, and this is the esoteric explanation for the marked improvement in health that is so often experienced by yoga students.

❑❑❑

7

STRETCHING FOR HEALTH AND BEAUTY

Yoga sessions are designed to be highly pleasurable experiences in which the movements are performed in relaxing, slow motion with very few repetitions, leaving you feeling elevated and revitalised, not drained.

Yoga and health are two words that are very closely related. The health benefits of yoga are widely known. Yoga is a popular aid in improving and attaining both physical and mental health. This is basically the most common reason why people practise yoga—for health reasons. They want to ease their back pain, find a method to ease stress, or ways to deal with their health problems.

Some poses stretch and align the body, while others primarily build muscle strength. Poses range from simple positions well suited to beginners, to very complicated and strenuous ones (such as head and shoulder stands) that should only be attempted by advanced practitioners.

In yoga, your own body weight acts as resistance. Depending on the position you are in, the poses engage different sets of muscles, which then get strengthened as you hold the pose. A big benefit of yoga is that it works every part of your body. In addition, it does not overwork certain muscles, so there is less chance of injury than with other types of exercise.

Beyond stretching and strengthening, some forms of yoga can also provide a good cardiovascular workout, especially those that have brisk movements of flow quickly from one pose into another.

While useful and satisfying on its own, yoga can also be a fine complement to other types of exercises. Certain poses, for instance, can be effective for stretching legs tightened by running, cycling, tennis or skiing or for releasing muscles stiffened by weight training.

Unlike stretching or fitness, yoga is more than just physical postures. Patanjali's eightfold path illustrates how the physical practice is just one aspect of yoga. Even within the physical practice, yoga is unique because we connect the movement of the body and the fluctuations of the mind to the rhythm of our breath. Connecting the mind, body and the breathe helps us to direct our attention inward. Through this process of inward attention, we learn to recognise our habitual thought patterns without labelling them, judging them or trying to change them. We become more aware of our experiences from moment to moment. The awareness that you cultivate is what makes yoga a practice rather than a task or a goal to be completed. Your body will most likely become much more flexible by doing yoga, and so will your mind.

Before doing the various asanas, it is essential to do exercises that loosen the stiff muscles. The stiffer you find yourself, the greater your need for the gentle stretching movements of yoga. A stiff, inflexible body cannot be a truly healthy and beautiful one. Remember that you must never strain, jerk or fight to achieve a more extreme position. Just go as far as you can, regardless of where it may be, and have the patience to hold as indicated.

The yogi attaches great value in terms of both health and beauty to a strong, elastic spine. An ancient yogic adage proclaims, "You are as young as your spine is flexible." Young people whose spines have grown rigid will appear to be much older than their actual years. Conversely, people who have retained the elasticity of their spines and limbs appear youthful and 'alive' in middle age and beyond.

"The body is the temple of the spirit, conceived in the image of its maker." This is the very first of the eternal truths that students must know so that each one becomes aware of the infinite power and beauty of his or her own, individual body. As this fact begins to penetrate the consciousness there is a natural attempt on the part of the students to cultivate those characteristics of beauty which lie within them.

It is important to perform the yoga movements with pose and balance, since these are essential qualities of beauty. There is something magnetic and radiant about the woman who moves, gestures, walks, sits and stands with natural grace and poise. She reflects an eternal aspect of true femininity. These movements must flow rhythmically and naturally from the centre of your being.

Pose, balance, grace and beautiful carriage emerge naturally from the yoga practice. Stiffness of the joints and limbs, a condition that inhibits poise and good posture, are eliminated through the stretching exercises. The slow motion, 'ballet-type' routine imparts a strong sense of rhythm and balance.

The following basic exercises will help you to unwind all the stiff muscles.

Neck

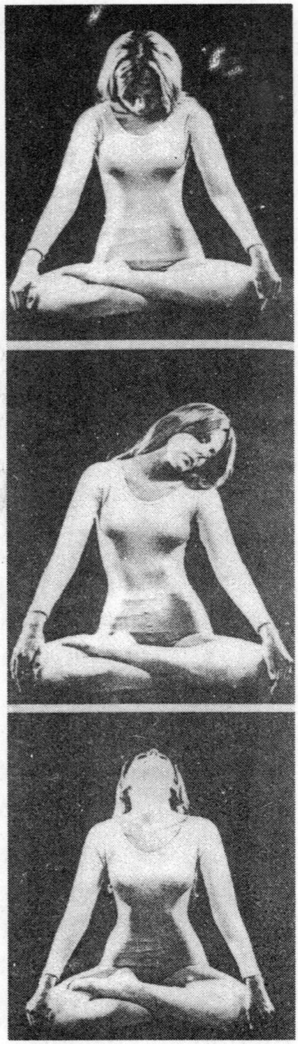

1. Sit in a cross-legged posture.
2. Bend head forward slowly, and rest chin against chest.
3. Sit erect.
4. Close eyes.
5. Hold for 10 counts.
6. Very slowly roll head to extreme left.
7. Hold to a count of 10.
8. Very slowly roll head to extreme backward position. Feel chin and throat muscles tightening.
9. Hold for 10 counts.
10. Very slowly roll head to extreme right.
11. Hold for 10 counts.
12. Very slowly roll head forward to position 1 Relax briefly.

Arms and Hands

1. Stand straight, feet together, hands by the sides.
2. Exhale, then begin deep inhalation (abdomen expands).

3. Simultaneously raise arms sideways and palms facing upward.
4. Continue deep inhalation, chest expands.
5. Bring hands to touch overhead.
6. Simultaneously raise high on toes.
7. Hold this position as steady as possible for a count of 5.
8. Begin deep exhalation, and very slowly lower to original position 1. Relax.
9. Clench and unclench 5 times your hands which are at the side of the body.

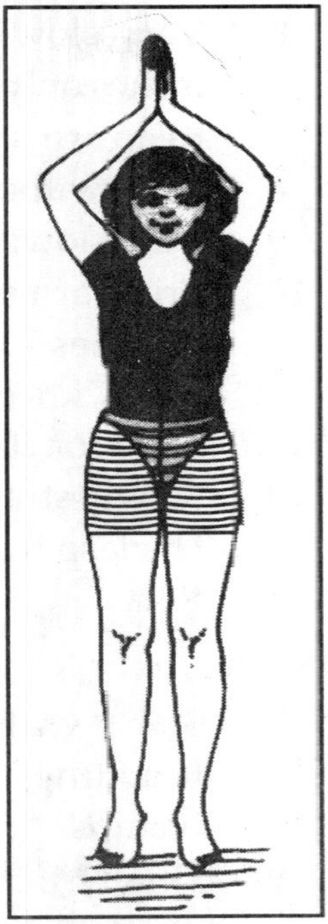

Chest

1. Stand in a relaxed posture, spine straight, arms at sides also feet close together.
2. Gracefully bring hands up to touch chest, palms facing outwards and downwards.
3. Slowly straighten arms outward in front at chest level. Feel elbows stretching.
4. Slowly bring arms behind you keeping them straight. Feel shoulders stretching.
5. Lower arms slightly so that fingers can be interlaced.

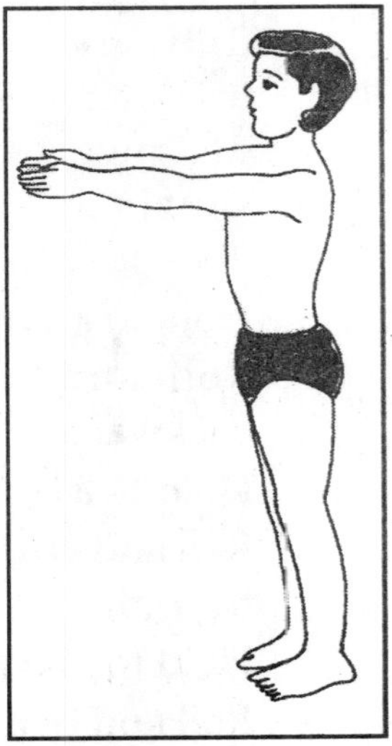

6. Very slowly and gently bend backward several inches only.
7. Keep arms high, look upward.
8. Hold without motion for 10 counts.
9. Very slowly and gently bend forward.
10. Bring arms over back and keep them high. Neck muscles are relaxed; forehead points towards knees, knees do not bend. Feel spine stretching.
11. Hold for 20 counts.
12. Slowly straighten up to upright position.
13. Unclasp hands.
14. Relax.

Waist

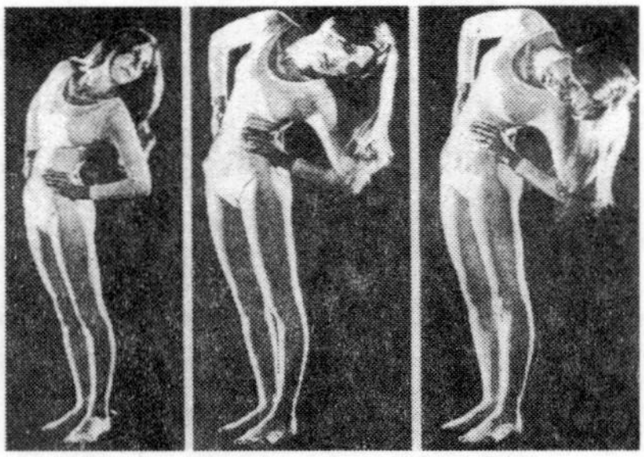

1. Stand with heels touching, hands on hips.
2. Slowly bend forward 30 degrees.
3. Roll and twist trunk a moderate distance to left slowly. Trunk does not bend to left, only the upper body.
4. Hold to a count of 5.
5. Roll and twist trunk a moderate distance backward.
6. Hold to a count of 5.
7. Roll and twist trunk slowly a moderate distance to the right.
8. Hold for 5 counts.
9. Roll and twist trunk forward to original position.

10. Hold for 5 counts.

Legs

1. Lie on your back, legs straight, hands spread sideways.
2. Bend right knee to chest.
3. Raise it up as straight as you can.
4. Slowly bring leg over the left leg, and attempt to touch the floor. Both shoulders remain on the floor. Bring leg as far as possible toward head, knee must not bend.
5. Hold to a count of 10.

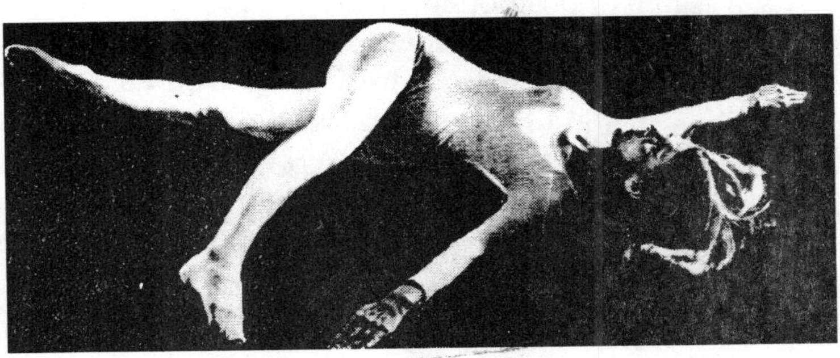

6. Bring right leg back to position 1.
7. Perform identical movements with left leg.
8. Hold for 10 counts.
9. Return to original position.
10. Relax.

❑❑❑

8

ASANAS

Yoga has simple and effective body movements that strengthen one's back, firm the stomach, and redistribute body weight. Yoga exercises stretch and tone the body muscles. They increase endurance and improve flexibility.

Yoga asanas or positions are the best among all exercises for toning muscles, lubricating joints and massaging the body. Yoga postures bring physical as well as mental, stability, health and vigour. These asanas were developed thousands of years ago, and have evolved over centuries. They work wonders in keeping the body healthy and the mind peaceful. Asanas exercise the nerves, glands ligaments and muscles. In other words, yoga exercises are the most comprehensive method of self-care.

Although asanas are very powerful, the effect becomes dramatic when they are done the right way. The mind must be in harmony with the body movements. For that, it is essential to equip yourself with the other tools of integral yoga.

Yoga has a range of poses and well set out sequences for persons with different profiles and conditions. There are several simple positions as well as more complex ones.

You must always begin with simple poses, and gradually over time move towards the complex ones. It is not as if maximum benefits cannot be achieved with simple positions. Quite contrarily, maximum benefits would be achieved by what is acceptable to your body.

To achieve the maximum benefits of yoga a specific yoga routine must be developed by first basic positions to free various rigid joints and get the mind in a suitable mode. Only then should you be moving to these positions. The process of yoga is just as important as the result. Asanas should be done with comfort, ease, alertness and steadiness, achieving a balance between ease and effort.

Asanas basically perform five foundations.

1. **Conative:** Conative action is the voluntary exercise of the organs of action. The asanas being the main yogic instrument of balancing the body, they consist of various physical postures which are designed to relieve tension.
2. **Cognitive:** The purpose of the asanas is to create a flow of positive energy so that our concentration is directed within ourselves, and the mind is able to perceive the effects of our purposive action. That is cognitive action.
3. **Mental:** When the earlier two actions are fused, our mind's discriminative faculty guides these organs to perform the asanas more correctly. The resultant rhythmic energy flow and awareness lead to a mental state of pure joy.
4. **Intellectual:** Physical postures, therefore, end up affecting the various interrelated channels of the mind-body complex. And ultimately the performance of perfect yogasana leads to the absolute intellectual absorption of the mind on a single task.

5. **Spiritual:** This in turn leads to the fusion of the individual spirit with the Divine Self.

Asana implies a posture in which one can remain steady, calm and comfortable, physically and mentally. According to Hindu legend there are 84,000 asanas for maintaining health, and Patanjali reduced them to 84 which are practised in India and abroad. In this book we shall discuss only the few that can be done without much effort.

Asanas must be practised regularly and punctually with faith, determination and tenacity, and without any interruptions or distractions. Asanas should be done with you wearing loose and comfortable clothes. Remove all unnecessary items, like shoes, belts, wallets, rings, etc., from the body.

Asanas should be done on an empty stomach, or at least two hours after a light meal. A folded blanket, or a soft carpet or rug on the floor is a must.

While doing the asanas care should be taken to breathe through the nose and not the mouth. After each asana, relax for a couple of minutes. After completing all the asanas, do the Shavasana (Corpse pose) for at least 10 minutes. This will soothe all the nerves, blood vessels, muscles, removing any strain, physical or mental.

Women who are pregnant or having their menstruation cycle should avoid doing these asanas during that period. Those suffering from certain ailments must practise the asanas only under the supervision of a qualified yoga teacher. It is better to avoid tobacco, smoking, liquor or opium.

And, most important of all, practice is what makes one perfect. As Patanjali said, "The young, the old, the extremely aged, even the sick and the infirm, obtain perfection in yoga by constant practice. Success in yoga is not obtained by more theoretical study or talking about it, or reading the sacred texts. Constant practice alone is the secret of its success."

Frequency of Practice

Yoga is amazing. Even if you only practise for one hour a week, you will experience the benefits of the practice. If you do more than that, you will certainly experience more benefits. You can start with two or three times a week for an hour or an hour and a half each time. If you can only do 20 minutes per session, that's fine too. Don't let time constraints or unrealistic goals be an obstacle. Do what you can and don't worry about it. You will likely find that after a while your desire to practise expands naturally and you will find yourself doing more and more.

Finding the Best Time to Practise

Your personal rhythm within a 24-hour period, as well as your relationship to the sun, moon, heat and cold, and the crispness or the thickness of the changing seasons, can indeed factor into which asanas you practise when. Some people are raring to go first thing in the morning, while other people won't even speak for at least an hour after the alarm goes off. Some love winter and outdoor activities such as skiing and snowboarding. Others put on a few pounds and hibernate in the winter, and come alive with the fire energy of July and August. Since an important part of yoga practice is getting to know yourself and how you change from moment to moment, it makes sense to let your energy inform you about how to practise according to the season or time of day. To begin, it is helpful to know that some poses are energising, and some are calming. For example, back bends are invigorating and not recommended before going to bed at night. Forward bends are calming and helpful when you are feeling over-stimulated. Surya namaskars or sun salutations create heat and flowing movement connected to the breath. Standing poses build strength, stamina, and a sense of grounding, since your feet are rooted into the earth. Balancing poses cultivate concentration, and twists detoxify the body and relieve tension in the head, neck and back. Inversion, which turn us upside down, literally changes our view of the world, and reminds us of the impermanent nature of everything, especially when we are stuck in a rut. In general, yoga practice is recommended in the morning or the early evening. A morning yoga session can be quite active, and consist of a full practice. Always finish with Shavasana (Corpse pose), no matter what time of day or season your practise. You may choose to do a different type of practice in the afternoon. While it can still be a complete practice, you may want to emphasise a series of seated forward bends, followed by a small back bend and simple twists. If you live in a place where it gets very hot in the summer, be mindful of the speed with which you move through your practices.

Categories of Yogasanas

Consummate mastery over the entire gamut of asanas is no doubt time-consuming, but what is of vital importance is the will to remain in the present moment and to let both the mind and body relax completely. Asanas harmonise our panic ability and mental energy flow by clearing any blockades in the subtle body leading to mental equilibrium and calmness. They make the mind strong, thus enabling our human body to suffer pain and unhappiness stoically and with fortitude.

The various categories of asanas are as follows:

1. Standing asanas
2. Forward bending asanas
3. Supine asanas
4. Inverted asanas
5. Abdominal and Lumbar asanas
6. Twisting asanas
7. Back bending asanas
8. Balancing asanas.

STANDING ASANAS

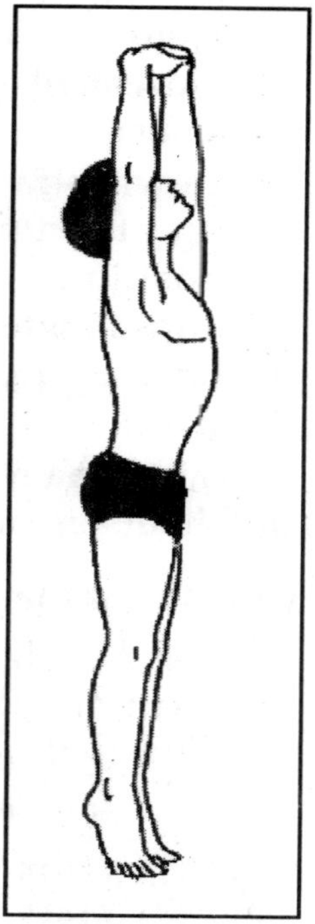

Beginners should start with these, as they bring elasticity in joints and muscles, and build up stamina and physical stability. This constitutes the most basic training in the early stages of yoga practice

Tadasana (Mountain Pose)

1. Stand on a mat and feet a few inches aprt.
2. Inhale deeply and slowly, and raise arms very slowly over head, elbows straight, and palms together.
3. Simultaneously raise high on toes, still inhaling.
4. Hold this position for 5 counts.
5. Begin deep exhalation and very slowly return to first position.
6. Relax.

Trikonasana (Triangle Pose)

1. Stand with legs approximately two feet apart.
2. Gracefully raise arms to shoulder level and palms facing downward.
3. Bend slowly to the left, keeping arms outstretched.
4. Take a firm hold on the ankle.
5. Slowly bring right arm up as far as possible.
6. Hold without movement for 15 counts.
7. Slowly straighten up to upright position, lower arms to sides, and bring legs together. Relax.

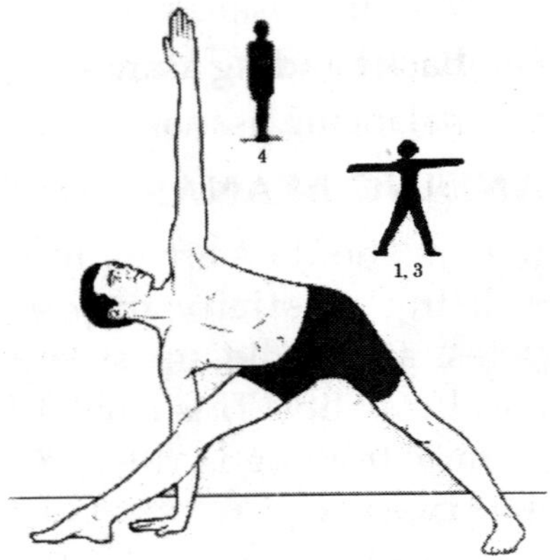

This asana relieves the pains in the joints of the neck and shoulders, and makes the spine flexible.

Padahastasana

1. Stand straight, feet slightly apart, arms by the sides.
2. Raise both arms, and slowly bend forward at the waist, knees firm, arms straight.
3. Slowly take the palms under the soles of the feet.
4. Slowly exhale while bending low.

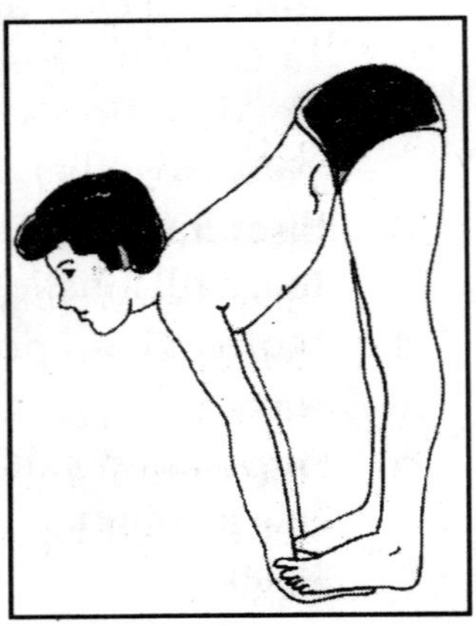

5. Put your forehead between the knees.
6. Hold this for 10 counts.
7. Gradually, return to original position. Relax.

This asana removes excess fat from the abdomen and waist.

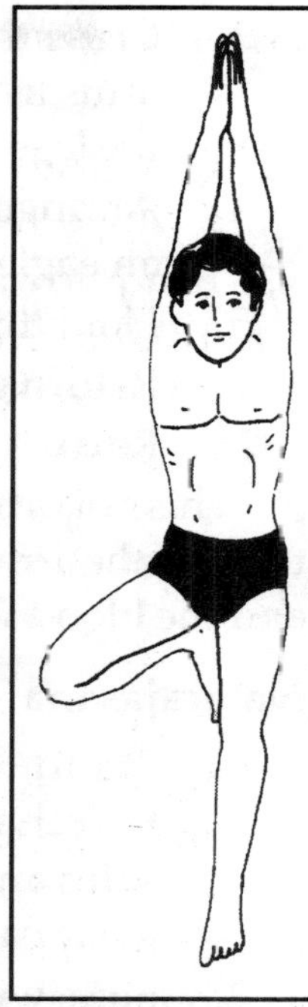

Vrukshasna (Tree Pose)

1. Stand on one leg.
2. Bend the other leg at the knee, and place its heel at the top of the inner thigh.
3. Join the palms and slowly raise the arms straight above the head, straightening the elbows.
4. Hold this to a count of 10.
5. Gradually return to the original position.
6. Repeat with the other leg.
7. Relax.

This asana helps strengthen the muscles of the legs and arms, as well as tones up the joints of the body.

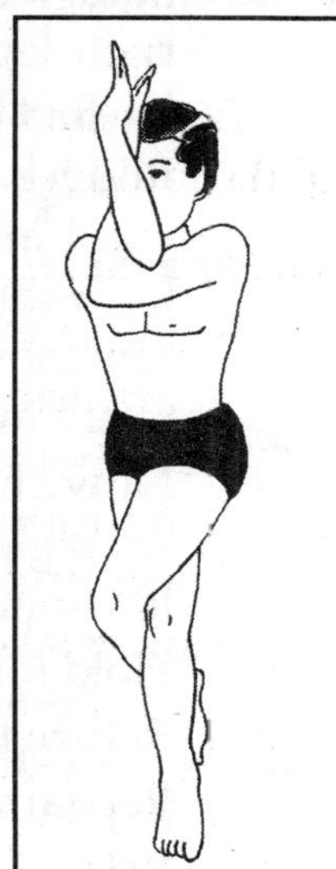

Garudasana (Eagle Pose)

1. Stand straight with feet together, hands by the sides.
2. Slowly take the left leg behind the right leg from the front, and let the left leg entwine the right leg.

3. Cross the arms at the elbows and keep the lower arms in front of the face, entwining each other as the legs.
4. Arrange the fingers in such a way as to resemble an eagle's beak, as shown in the figure.
5. Hold this pose for a count of 20.
6. Return gradually to the first position.
7. Relax.

This helps to strengthen the leg and thigh muscles and those of the arms as well. It helps to relieve rheumatic pains, and the blood vessels are stretched.

Natarajasana

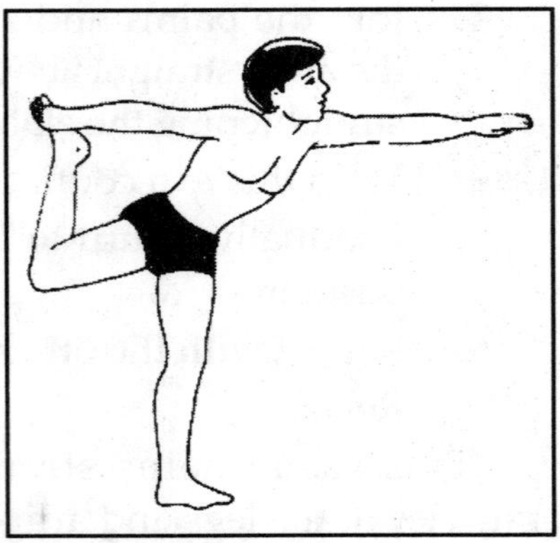

1. Stand with heels together, arms at sides and right arm overhead.
2. Shift weight to the right leg, and raise left foot behind you.
3. Reach back with left hand and hold the left foot. The right arm moves forward to aid in keeping the balance.
4. Now, holding the right arm straight ahead at an angle of 45 degrees and raise the left foot up as illustrated.
5. Hold for 10 counts.
6. Return to original position.
7. Repeat with the other leg.
8. Relax.

5. Put your forehead between the knees.
6. Hold this for 10 counts.
7. Gradually, return to original position. Relax.

This asana removes excess fat from the abdomen and waist.

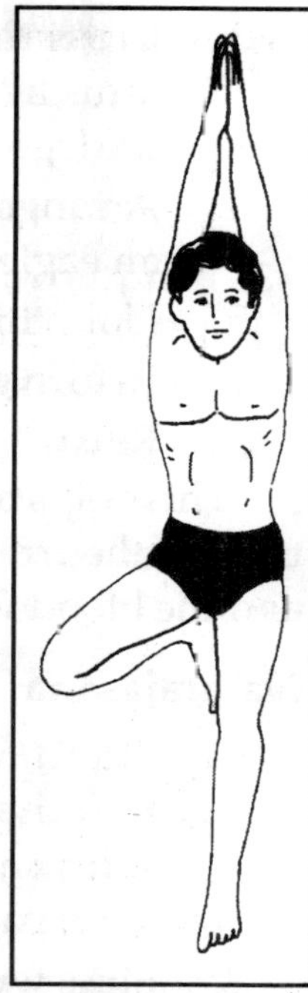

Vrukshasna (Tree Pose)

1. Stand on one leg.
2. Bend the other leg at the knee, and place its heel at the top of the inner thigh.
3. Join the palms and slowly raise the arms straight above the head, straightening the elbows.
4. Hold this to a count of 10.
5. Gradually return to the original position.
6. Repeat with the other leg.
7. Relax.

This asana helps strengthen the muscles of the legs and arms, as well as tones up the joints of the body.

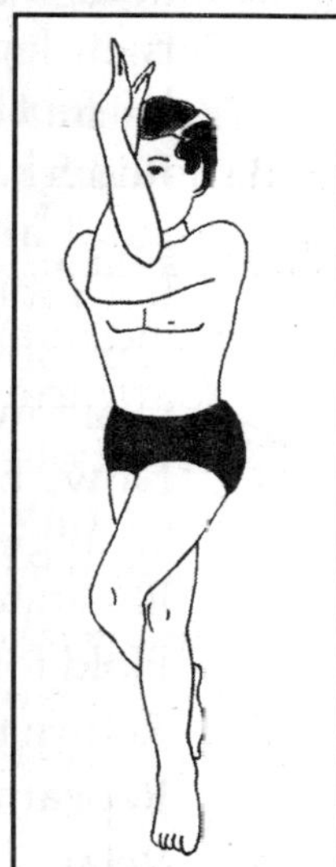

Garudasana (Eagle Pose)

1. Stand straight with feet together, hands by the sides.
2. Slowly take the left leg behind the right leg from the front, and let the left leg entwine the right leg.

3. Cross the arms at the elbows and keep the lower arms in front of the face, entwining each other as the legs.
4. Arrange the fingers in such a way as to resemble an eagle's beak, as shown in the figure.
5. Hold this pose for a count of 20.
6. Return gradually to the first position.
7. Relax.

This helps to strengthen the leg and thigh muscles and those of the arms as well. It helps to relieve rheumatic pains, and the blood vessels are stretched.

Natarajasana

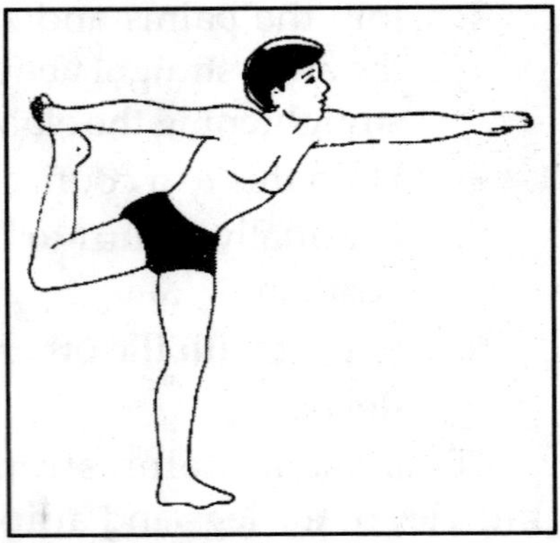

1. Stand with heels together, arms at sides and right arm overhead.
2. Shift weight to the right leg, and raise left foot behind you.
3. Reach back with left hand and hold the left foot. The right arm moves forward to aid in keeping the balance.
4. Now, holding the right arm straight ahead at an angle of 45 degrees and raise the left foot up as illustrated.
5. Hold for 10 counts.
6. Return to original position.
7. Repeat with the other leg.
8. Relax.

This asana exercises all the joints of the body, and makes the waist flexible.

Ardha Chakrasana (Half Wheel Pose)

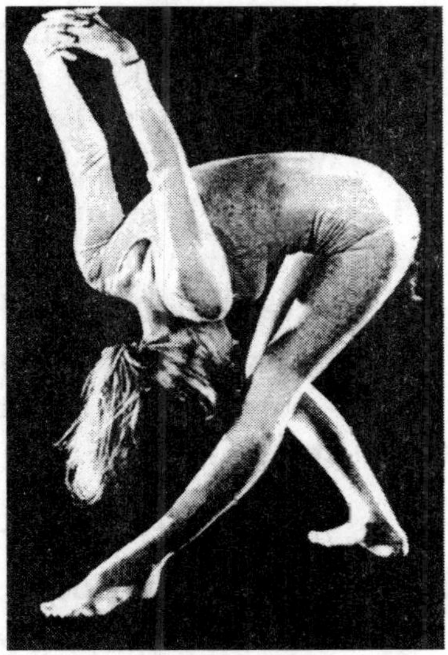

1. Stand in a relaxed posture, spine straight, arms at sides, feet close together.
2. Gracefully bring hands up to touch chest, palms facing outward.
3. Slowly straighten arms outward at chest level in front, feel elbows stretching.
4. Slowly bring arms behind you, keeping them as high as you can. Feel shoulders stretching.
5. Lower arms slightly, so that fingers can be interlaced. Do not bend trunk at this point.
6. Very slowly and gently bend backward several inches only. Keep arms high, look upward.
7. Hold to 10 counts.
8. Very slowly and gently bend forward, arms high over back, neck muscles relaxed, face parallel to the ground. Knees do not bend. Feel spine stretching gently.
9. Hold for 20 counts.
10. Bend the body more so that the head is as close to the knees as possible, with the hand still clasped,

raised as high back as possible. Hold for 5 counts.

11. Straighten up slowly, hands still back.
12. Extend your left leg to the side and front.
13. Bend forward once again slowly.
14. Twist trunk slightly to the left, and bring the head close to the knee, left knee still straight, right knee slightly bent. Feel stretching of the hamstring muscles.
15. Hold to 10 counts.
16. Straighten to upright position and bring left leg in.
17. Extend right leg and repeat the process.
18. Relax upon completion.

These movements help to develop and firm your chest and bust.

SITTING ASANAS

Padmasana (Lotus Pose)

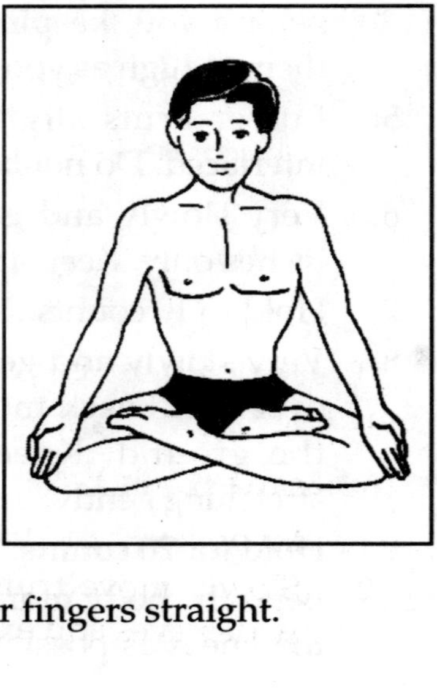

1. Sit on mat, legs extended and hands on lap.
2. Hold the right foot and place it on the left thigh.
3. Then hold the left foot and place it on the right thigh.
4. Place the hands on the knees.
5. Let the tip of each thumb touch the tip of the index finger, other fingers straight.

6. Stay in this position, eyes closed, for 2 minutes, which can later be increased when you go into meditation.

This asana is useful for Pranayama and self-realisation.

Paschimottanasana

1. Sit with legs stretched out, hands on knee and feet together.
2. Raise arms slowly to shoulder level, inhaling as you do.
3. Gracefully bend forward, keeping arms outstretched.
4. Hold the feet with your hands, and touch the knees with the forehead.
5. Keep this position to a count of 20.
6. Slowly exhale the return to the original position.
7. Relax.

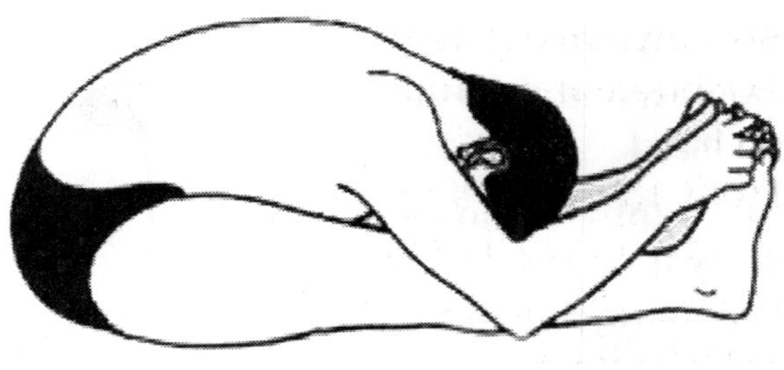

This helps to stretch your back, toning up the abdominal muscles.

Simhasana (Lion Pose)

1. Sit on heels and hands resting on knees.
2. Slowly move trunk forward and simultaneously widen eyes and extend tongue.

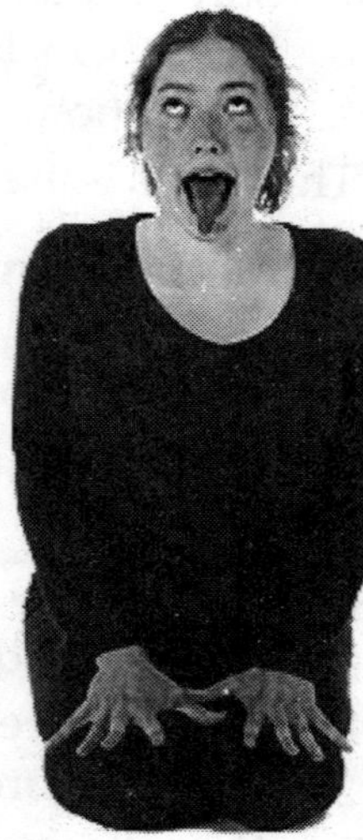

3. Spread the fingers apart on the knees. You can feel the pull of muscles of the face and neck. Open your mouth and bring the tongue out as far as possible.
4. Hold for 15 counts.
5. Slowly withdraw tongue and relax eyes and fingers.
6. Relax.

This asana helps to firm the muscle of the face and neck.

Gomukhasana (Cow Face Pose)

1. Sit in a cross-legged posture.
2. Place left hand on the centre of your back, palm outward.

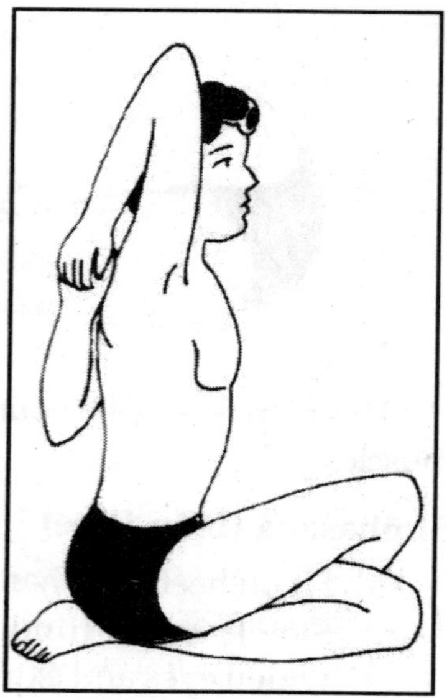

3. Bring right hand over shoulder and clasp the left hand.
4. Pull right arm down an inch or two. Feel the intense pull in the right shoulder.
5. Hold for 5 counts.
6. Reverse the arm positions and continue the movements.
7. Hold for 5 counts.
8. Relax

This asana helps to loosen the shoulder muscles and improves your posture.

Ardha Matsyendrasana

1. Extend legs straight outward.
2. Place right sole against left thigh.
3. Take a firm hold on the left ankle, and swinging it over the right knee and place the sole on the floor.
4. Place left hand on floor behind you.
5. Now bring the right arm over left knee and take a firm hold of left foot.

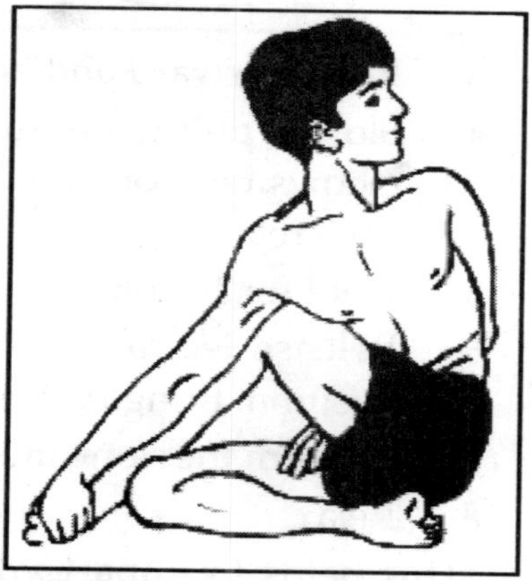

6. Slowly twist trunk and head as far to the left as possible.
7. Move the left hand around back and hold right side of the waist and chin close to the shoulder.
8. Hold for 10 counts.
9. Lower hand to floor, turn trunk and head forward, and return to original position.
10. Relax.

This helps in immediately loosening the entire spinal column.

Janu Shirasana

1. Sit with legs outstretched before you.
2. Place sole of right foot firmly against the upper inside of the left thigh.

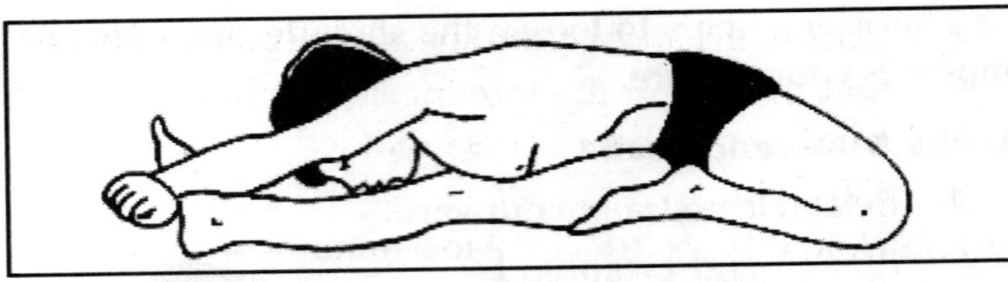

3. Reach forward and hold left foot firmly.
4. Slowly pull trunk downward as far as possible, elbows bent outward, forehead toward knee and neck relaxed.
5. Hold for 10 counts.
6. Release leg and slowly straighten into upright position. Bringing the hands to rest on the knees.
7. Perform the same movements with the right foot.
8. Relax.

This helps to impart youthful spring to legs, while loosening the back muscles.

Siddhasana (Half Lotus Pose)

1. Sit down with both legs straight out.
2. Bend the left knee, and place the heel of the left foot against the right inside thigh near the genitals.
3. Bend the right knee and place the right foot over the left, so that the heel of the right foot touches the genitals.

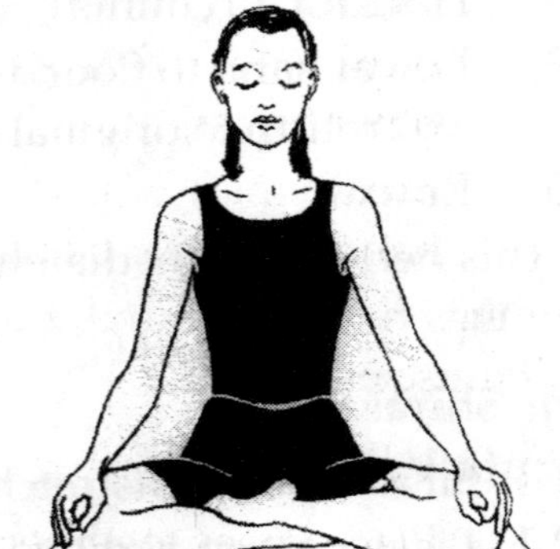

4. Place both hands on the knees, with palms outward.
5. Join the tips of the forefinger and thumb of each hand, with other fingers extended.
6. Close your eyes.
7. Hold this position for 2 to 5 minutes.
8. Relax.

Relieves stiffness in the joints

KNEELING ASANAS

Vajrasana (Thunderbolt Pose)

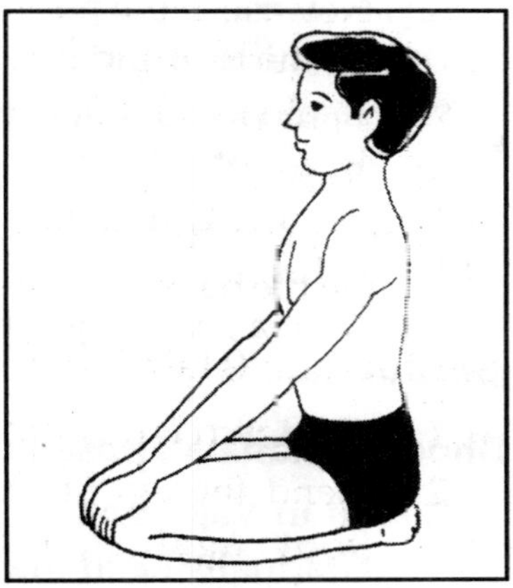

1. Kneel down.
2. Rest the buttocks on the ground between the feet, with toes pointing backward.
3. Stretch the hands and place the wrists on the knees, palm facing out.
4. Join the tips of the thumb and forefinger, while keeping the other fingers straight.
5. Breathe slowly and rhythmically several times (the hands can also be kept holding the knees).

This helps in stimulating digestion, and exercises the calf muscles.

Supta Vajrasana

1. Place knees together and slowly sit back on heels.
2. Place fingertips on floor at your sides.

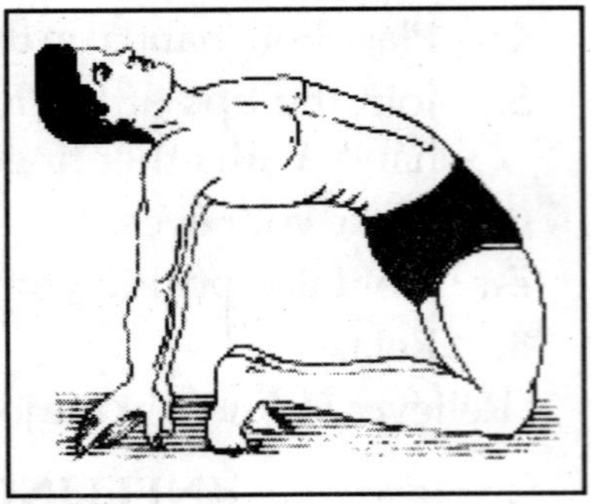

3. Move arms slowly backward until you can rest your hands on the floor in the position illustrated.
4. Lower head backward slowly as far as possible.
5. Simultaneously arch spine.
6. Slowly return to original position.
7. Now raise the heel from the floor resting the body on the toes and ball of the feet.
8. Again lean backward as explained before. Hold for 10 counts.
9. Gradually return to original position.
10. Relax.

This asana helps in giving flexibility to your feet, ankles and toes.

Bhoo Namana Vajrasana (Yoga Mudra)

1. Sit in Vajrasana.
2. Gradually bend the body forward.
3. Lock the arms at the back of the body.
4. Inhale, and slowly exhale, stretching the neck downward so that the nose touches the ground.
5. Hold for 10 counts.
6. Return to original position.
7. Relax.

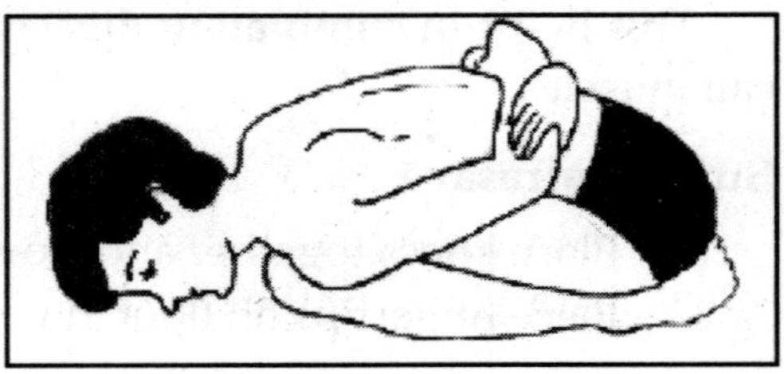

This increases the elasticity of the spine, and strengthens the muscles of the abdomen and the chest.

Ushtrasana (Camel Pose)

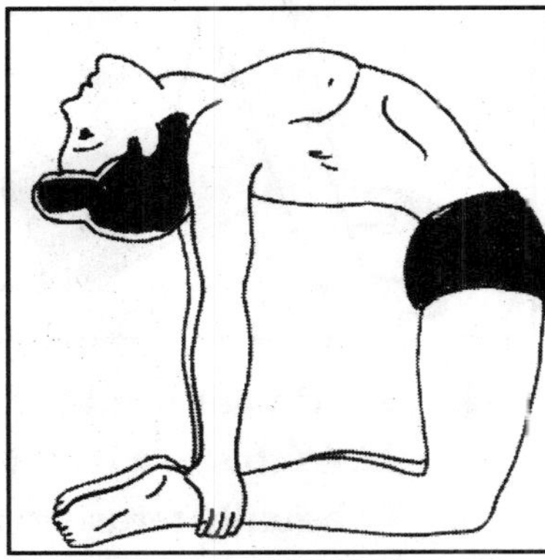

1. Sit in Vajrasana, leaving a gap of 15 cms between the knees, and between the heels.
2. Breathing deeply in, place your hands on your waist.
3. Slowly bend your head backward.
4. Bend back from your waist.
5. Gradually bring your hands from your waist to your ankles and hold them.
6. Stay to a count of 15.
7. Return to normal position.
8. Relax.

This helps to trim the waist and tone the muscles of the back.

ABDOMINAL ASANAS

Bhujangasana (Cobra Pose)

1. Lie on the mat; face downwards, arms by the sides, forehead on the floor.
2. Gracefully place hands beneath shoulders, fingers pointing outward.
3. Gradually raise the trunk from waist upward, straightening the elbows.

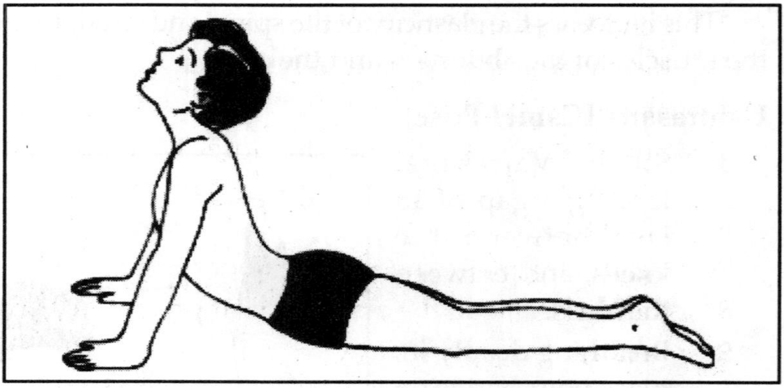

4. Bend your head backward as far as possible.
5. Hold this to a count of 10.
6. Gradually return to the original position.
7. Relax.

This helps to remove all tension from your back and spine.

Dhanurasana (Bow Pose)

1. Lie on your stomach, chin on the floor, arms at sides.

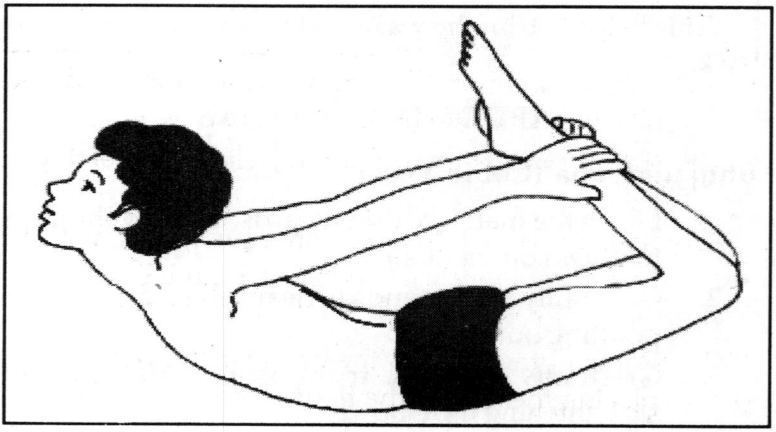

2. Bend knees and bring feet forward.
3. Reach back and attempt to hold feet.
4. Slowly raise trunk.
5. Simultaneously raise the knees, head bent backward.
6. Hold to a count of 10.
7. Gradually lower knees to the floor.
8. Return slowly to the original position.
9. Relax.

This asana helps to firm flabby areas of your back.

Mayurasana (Peacock Pose)

1. Sit on your knees, with the knees slightly apart.
2. Place the palms on the floor in between the knees, the fingers pointing backward.

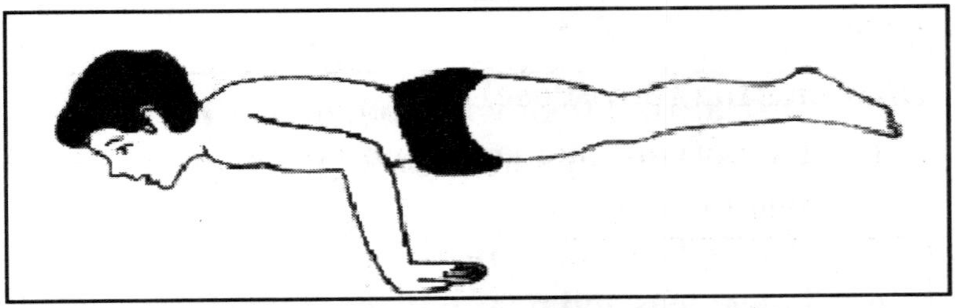

3. Gradually bring the elbows close to the abdomen just below the navel.
4. Resting the diaphragm on the elbows, stretch your legs.
5. Balance the whole body on your palms, with the trunk and feet above the floor, parallel to it.
6. Hold to a count of 5.
7. Return gradually to the original position, by first placing the feet on the floor.

8. Relax.

This helps to strengthen the muscles in the hands and arms.

Shalabhasana (Locust Pose)

1. Rest ball of chin on floor.
2. Place fists, thumbs down, firmly against floor at sides.

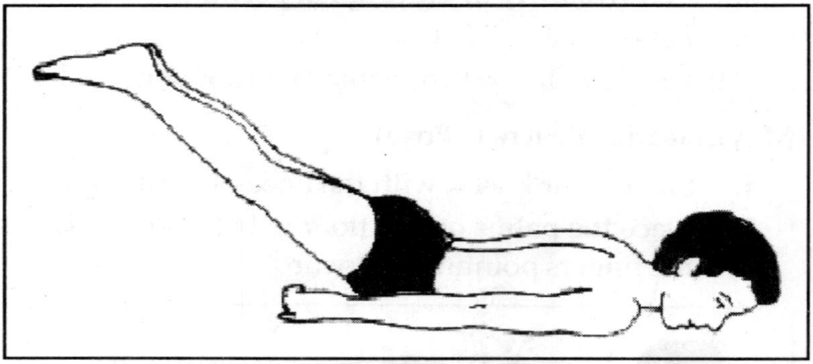

3. Push against floor with both fists.
4. Raise both legs at high as possible, the knees slightly bent.
5. Hold to a count of 10.
6. Lower legs and relax with cheek on floor.

This helps to firm your legs and tones up the abdominal muscles.

Konasana

1. Keeping the feet close together, sit on the floor.
2. Place the palms on the floor at the side, fingers pointing backward.
3. Keeping the arms perpendicular to the shoulder, extend the legs.

4. Inhale deeply, and balance your body on your palms and heel, head bent back. The elbows and knees should not be bent.
5. Hold to a count of 10.

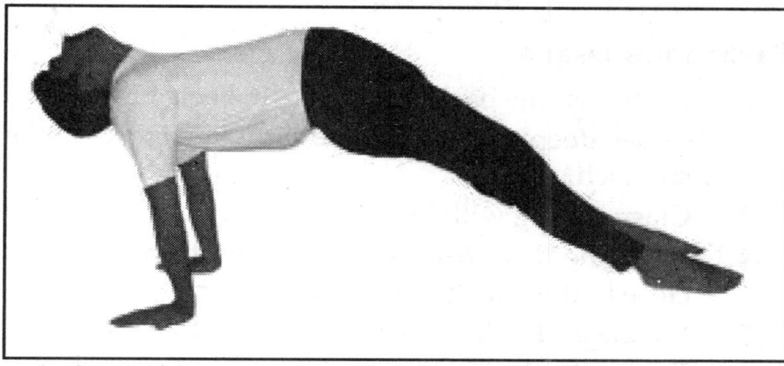

6. Slowly lower the body to the floor and return to the original position.
7. Relax.

This strengthens the muscles of the shoulders.

Bhadrasana

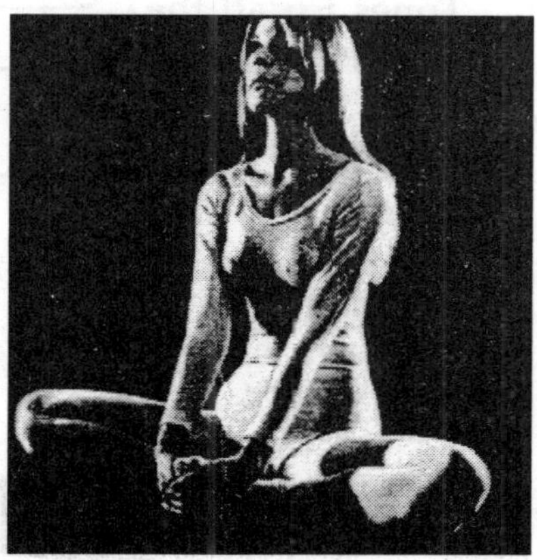

1. In a seated position, clasp feet firmly.
2. Pull heels in as far as possible, sitting erect.
3. Pull up against feet, and slowly lower knees, feel thighs tightening.
4. Pull hard against feet.
5. Hold to a count of 20.

6. Relax hold on feet and let knees be raised.
7. Relax.

This asana helps in firming up your thighs.

SPINE ASANAS

Pavanamuktasana

1. Lie flat on the back, legs straight, heels together.
2. Inhale deeply and bend the right knee toward the stomach.
3. Clasp the leg with both hands.
4. Raise the head from the floor, and bring the chin close to the knee to touch it.
5. Exhale and hold to 10 counts.
6. Return to the original position.
7. Relax.
8. Repeat with the other leg.

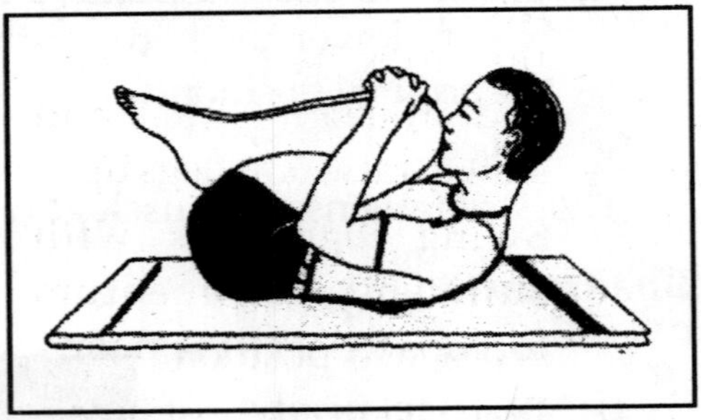

Tones up all the muscles of the body.

Uttanapadasana

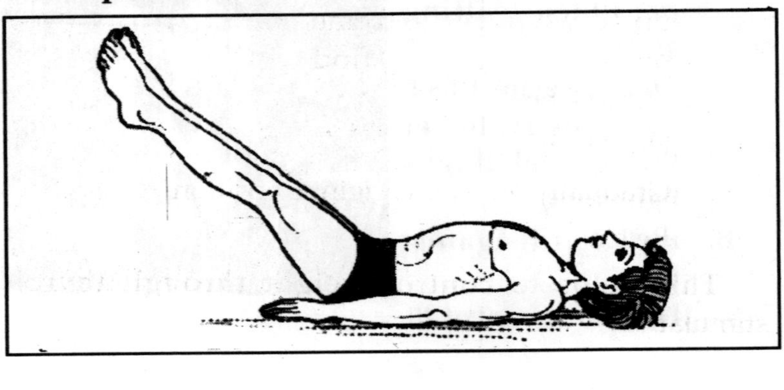

1. Lie on your back, legs straight, hands by the side, heels together.
2. Inhaling slowly, lift both legs up slowly to 45 degrees.
3. Hold this to 8 counts.
4. Exhaling, bring the feet down slowly.
5. Relax.

This helps in removing excess fat from the body, while toning up the thigh muscles.

Vilomasana

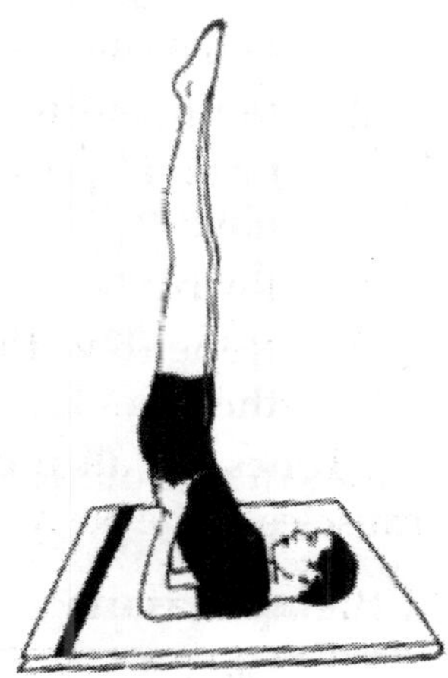

1. Lie flat on your back, hands on the side.
2. Brace palms against the floor, tense leg and abdominal muscles, and slowly raise both legs up.
3. Swing legs back with sufficient momentum for hips to leave the floor.
4. Brace hands against hips.
5. Very slowly straighten up to whatever extreme position you find comfortable.
6. Hold to 10 counts.
7. Gradually return to original position.
8. Relax.

This helps to control weight through thyroid stimulation.

Sarvangasana

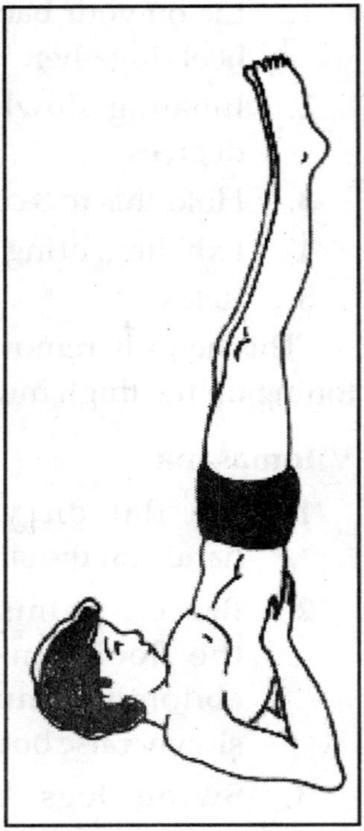

1. Lie flat on your back, hands by the side.
2. Inhale and slowly raise both legs together.
3. Then raise the legs, hips and trunk with the hands supporting the back on two sides, upper arm and elbows on ground.
4. Raise the body till the legs, hips and trunk are in a vertical position.
5. Look at the toes of the feet.
6. Hold to a count of 5, and then return very gradually to the original position.
7. Relax.

Halasana (Plough Pose)

1. Lying on back, brace palms against the floor and raise the legs.

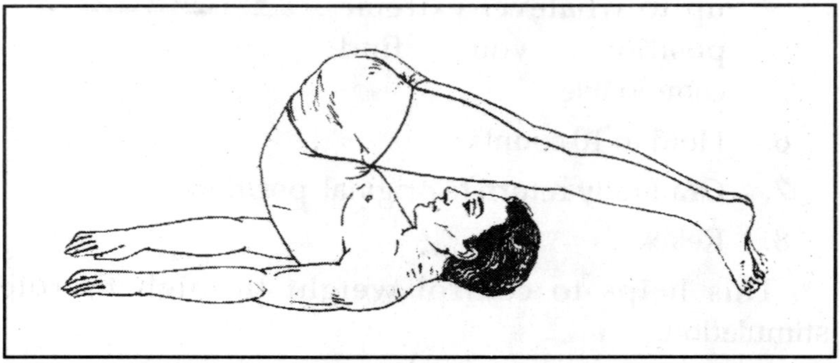

2. Push against the floor with hands and swing legs back as slowly as possible.
3. Continue to move trunk upward and slowly lower legs to floor, keeping knees straight and let the toes touch the floor.
4. Hold to a count of 5.
5. Return slowly to the original position.
6. Relax.

Helps to strengthen and manipulate your spine.

Uttitha Merudandasana

1. Lie on left side, legs together, head supported by left hand, right hand firmly on floor.
2. Very slowly raise the right leg as high as possible.
3. Hold for a count of 10.
4. Pushing firmly against the floor with the hand, raise both legs a short distance, legs remaining together.
5. Hold to a count of 5.
6. Lower slowly to the floor.
7. Repeat, lying on the right side.
8. Relax.

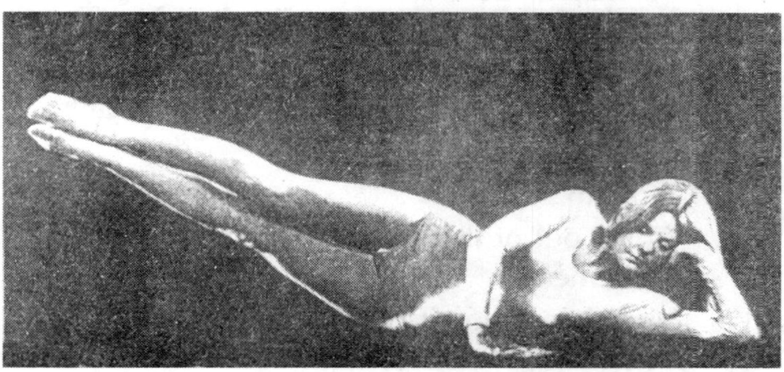

This is powerful movement for the hips and abdomen.

Shirshasana (Head Stand Pose)

This posture is performed with the aid of a small pillow or cushion.

1. Seated on heels, interlace fingers.
2. Place hands firmly on pillow.
3. Place top of head on pillow. Cradle back of head and hold head in clasped hands; rest toes on floor.
4. Push toes against floor and raise body as illustrated.
5. Very slowly, inch forward with toes, and bring bent knees as close to chest as possible.
6. Place your complete weight on head and arms straighten back.
7. Push lightly against floor with toes; slowly bring body into position as illustrated.

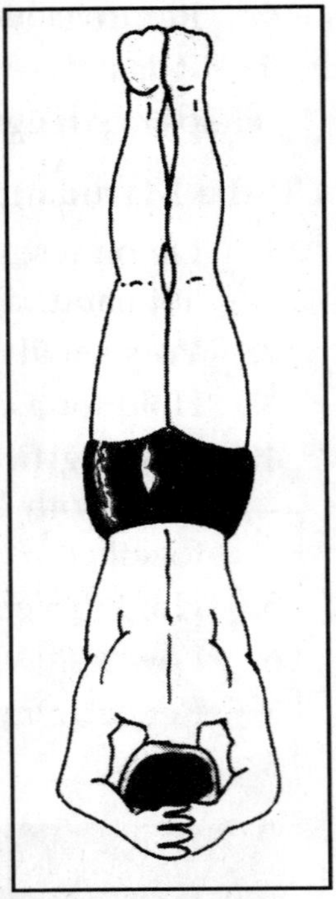

8. In very slow motion and with complete control straighten your legs, maintaining the balance of your body on head and arms.
9. Hold to 10 counts.
10. Come out of this posture slowly by reversing the movements.
11. Keep knees close to chest.
12. Lower legs slowly, with control. Do not come

crashing down with feet banging against the floor.

13. Rest in head down position, knees on the floor, toes on the floor keep to a count of 20.
14. Relax.

Shavasana (Death Pose)

1. Lie flat on your back, legs straight, and hands by the sides', palms up.
2. Keep the eyes closed, and breathe deeply.
3. Begin by consciously and gradually relaxing each part and muscle of the body, from the toes to the feet, calves, knees, thighs, abdomen, hips, back, chest, fingers, neck, face and head.
4. Inhale and exhale slowly and deeply.
5. Direct your attention to your breathing and gradually to God.
6. Remain relaxed for 10-15 minutes.

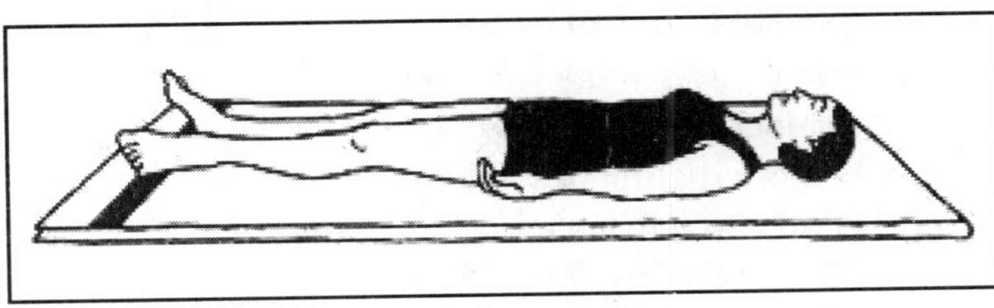

OTHER ASANAS

Veerasana (Warrior Pose)

1. Sit on the floor, spine straight, eyes ahead.
2. Bend the left leg, and place the heel below the anus.
3. Bend the other leg at the knee, and place it on the thigh of the left leg.
4. Raise your arms up and bring them together, resting them on the hand, palms together.

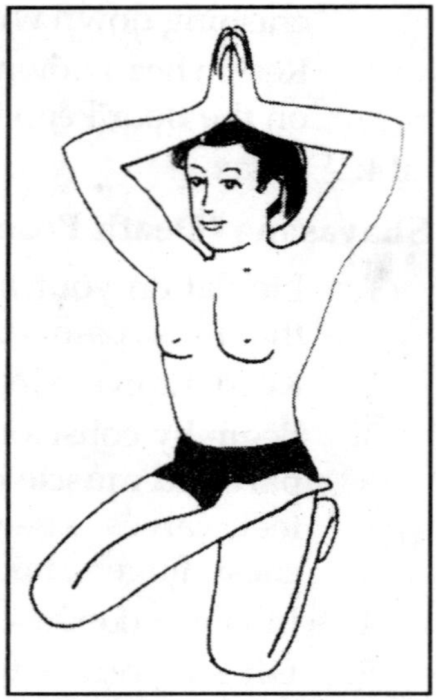

5. Breathe slowly, and hold this position to 8 counts.
6. Return to the original position.
7. Reverse the movements of the legs.
8. Relax.

This asana helps in breath control and tones up the leg muscles.

Parshvakonasana (Side Angle Pose)

1. Stand straight, feet together and hands by the sides.
2. Take one of the legs sideways to keep a distance of three to four feet between the feet.
3. Inhale, and raise the arms sideways, keeping it parallel to the ground.
4. While exhaling, turn the right leg toward the left.
5. Bend the left knee till the thigh is parallel to the ground and right leg straight.

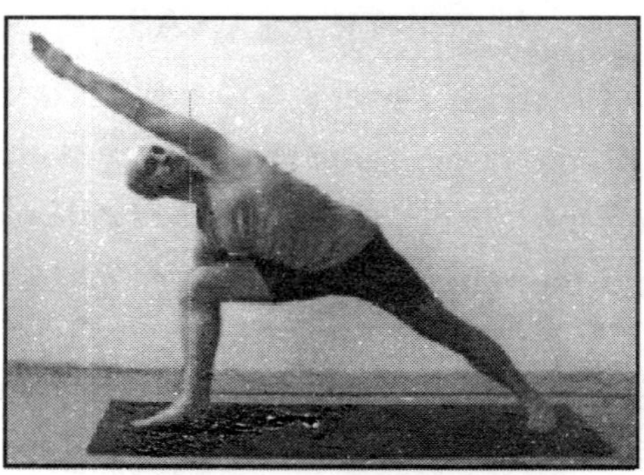

6. Press the left hand palm on the floor beside the left foot.
7. Bring the right arm over the front, and stretch it straight above the right ear. The arm should be parallel to the ground.
8. Raise the head and look at the tips of the right hand fingers.
9. Hold this position to 10 counts.
10. Return to original position.
11. Reverse the movements with the other leg and arm.
12. Relax.

Removes stiffness in the neck joint and knee joints, and reduces the fat around the waist and hips.

Supta Padangushthasana

1. Lie flat on your back, legs stretched and hands by the sides.
2. While inhaling slowly, lift the right leg slowly, and bring it straight up, perpendicular to the ground.
3. Rest the left hand on the left thigh.
4. As you exhale, hold the right foot big toe with the right hand.

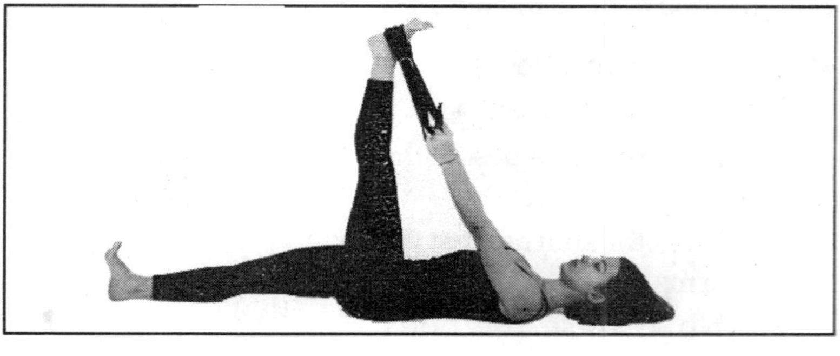

5. Simultaneously, pull the head backward, resting the crown on the ground.
6. Hold to a count of 10, breathing normally.
7. Exhale, and bring the right leg over the left leg, still holding the big toe.
8. Turn the head in the opposite direction.
9. Hold to a count of 10.
10. Return to the original position.
11. Relax.

Helps to strengthen and tone the muscles of the legs, thighs and arms.

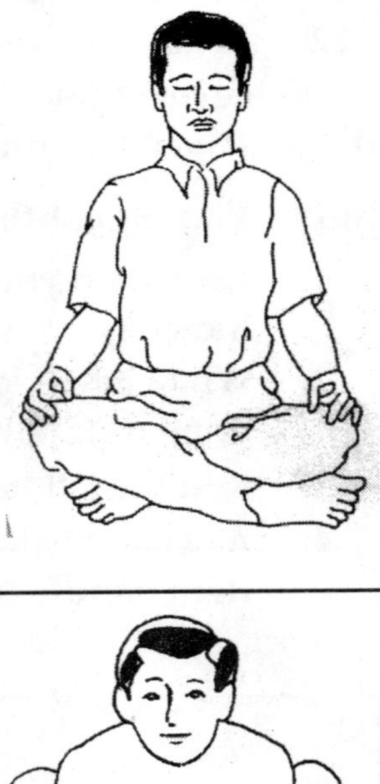

Sukhasana (Pleasure Pose)

1. Sit cross-legged comfortably on a mat.
2. Keep your back straight.
3. With head straight, either gaze ahead or close your eyes.
4. Keep your hands loosely on your laps.

This is an easy pose and very comfortable to be in at all times.

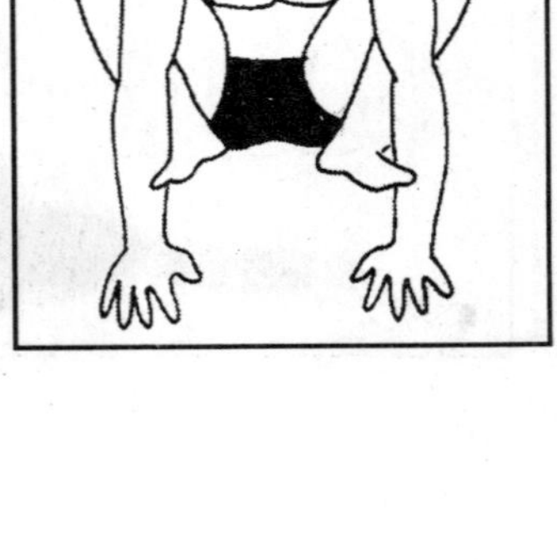

Bakasana (Crane Pose)

1. Sit on your heels, palms on the ground beside the left.
2. Press the shin against the arms.
3. Now, raise the body

from the ground, balancing on the hands.

4. Cross the legs at the feet, the right sole on the left foot.
5. Hold this position to a count of 10.
6. Lower the body gradually to the ground.
7. Relax.

This strengthens the muscles of the abdomen and spine, as well as the arms and hands.

Naukasana (Boat Pose)

1. Sit straight on the mat, legs stretched out, and hands by the side.
2. Hold the back of the head.
3. Inhale deeply, then as you slowly exhale, lean back a little and simultaneously raise the legs from the floor to about 30 degrees, balancing the body on the buttocks.
4. Hold this to a count of 10.
5. Now stretch the hands straight in front on the side

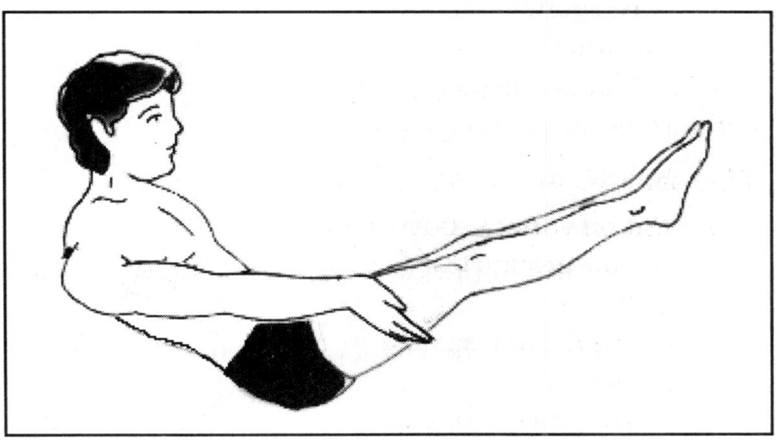

of the knees, keeping the arms parallel to the ground.

6. Hold to 5 counts.
7. Return slowly to the original position.
8. Relax.

This asana helps in toning up and strengthening the back.

Urvasana (Dancer's Pose)

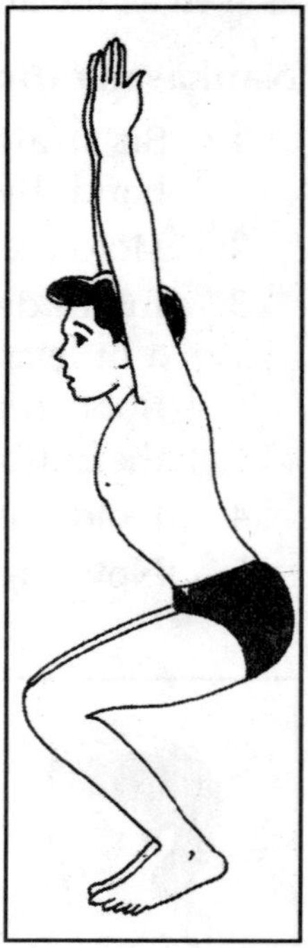

1. Stand with heels together.
2. Place palms together on top of head. Elbows are parallel with sides.
3. In very slow motion bend knees and lower body, balancing the body on toes, heels raised from the floor.
4. Continue to lower into the squatting posture.
5. Without pause, begin to push up very slowly.
6. Straighten into upright position, remaining on toes.
7. Lower soles of feet to floor.
8. Relax.

Kandharasana (Back Push-Up)

1. Lie on the floor, knees together and bent, heels drawn.
2. Rest the palms on the floor, close to the head.
3. Push against floor with hands and feet.

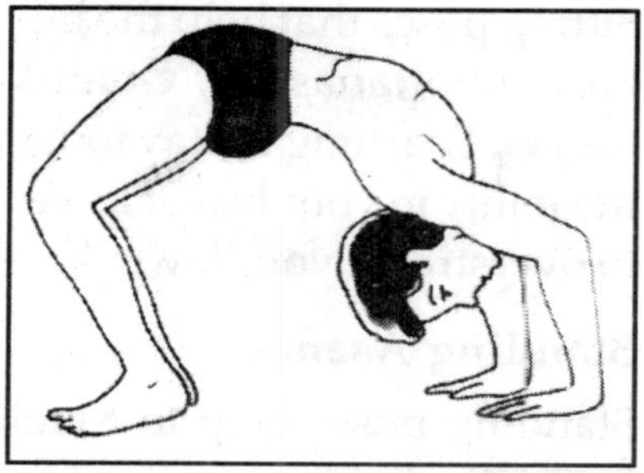

4. Raise body a moderate distance.
5. Hold to a count of 5.
6. Raise the body higher as far as possible, keeping knees together.
7. Hold to 10 counts.
8. Slowly lower body to the floor.
9. Relax.

BENEFITS OF ASANAS

Sitting Asanas

Sitting cross-legged is an important part of yoga practice, and is commonly used breathing and meditation practices. It requires flexibility in the back thighs, back of the pelvis, the inner thighs, as well as external rotation of the hip joints. These are all very strong muscles that can take a long time to stretch. Whether you sit in a simple cross-legged posture like Sukhasana or a more difficult pose like Padmasana, developing the flexibility to sit easily is a gradual process.

And it is important to note that all have a different anatomical structures in their hips, which may potentially inhibit this kind of movement. If this is the case for you, then trying to work up to Padmasana is an inappropriate goal. Try other poses that may be more comfortable, like Vajrasana, sitting on your heels, Veerasana, sitting between your heels or Gomukhasana. If you have difficulty maintaining an erect spine while sitting cross-legged, begin by sitting on the edge of a cushion, bolster or rolled blanket.

Sitting poses that help the hip muscles are Janu Shirshana, Paschimottanasana, Gomukhasana, Ardha Matsyendrasana. Learning to stay longer in these poses will help the flexibility in your hips. However you need to be careful not to overstretch your lower back.

Standing Asanas

Standing poses help to toughen up the leg muscles and loosen the tightness around the hips. Parshvakonasana and Veerasana are excellent for this purpose.

Spine Asanas

Supta Padanushthasana and Dhanurasana are good for your hips to gradually open up and give them flexibility.

❑❑❑

9

SURYA NAMASKAR (Sun Salutation)

The Sanskrit word 'Surya' means 'Sun'. 'Namaskar' is the Hindi word for 'Namaste', from the root *Nam* (to Bow). Namaskar means salutation, salute, greeting or praise.

All sessions of yoga asanas begin with Surya Namaskar, or Sun Salutation. In Hindu mythology, the sun god is worshipped as a symbol of health and immortal life. The *Rig Veda* declares, "Surya is the soul, both the moving and unmoving beings." The sun salutation originated as a series of prostrations to the sun. Traditionally, it is performed at dawn, facing the rising sun.

Surya Namaskar is not a formal part of traditional Hathayoga, though it is composed of a series of twelve yoga asanas performed in sequence. However, it is of so much value that it has now been accepted as a part of Hathayoga. In fact, many people use it as a warm-up before the asana practice. If there is a shortage of time, some people just do Surya Namaskar in lieu of the actual asana practice, and still derive substantial benefit. It is typically performed in the open air, facing the sun, at sunrise, when Surya, the life generator, is invoked by this yogic exercise.

Surya Namaskar limbers up the whole body in preparation for the yogasanas. It is a graceful sequence of 12 yoga postures performed as one continuous exercise. Each posture counteracts the one before, stretching the body in a different way, and alternately expanding and outreaching the chest to regulate the breathing.

The series of flowing movement's synchronise with the breath. This excellent warm-up exercise consists of a sequence of positions that move the spine in various ways and promote flexibility in the limbs. It is of special benefit to beginners to stiff people, and to the elderly, since it helps the body to gain flexibility. It also regulates the breath and focuses the mind.

Surya Namaskar is considered as the best exercise for the human body. It consists of important yogasanas and pranayama. The pranayama and thus its advantages are skilfully incorporated in Surya Namaskar. The mantras (Beeja Mantras), which are chanted before practising, are also very helpful. Surya Namaskar is the best way to burn the calories and reduce weight. It is often recommended for obesity.

The full cycle of 12 poses make one round. You can start with as many rounds as you can do, without getting out of breath. Try to work up your way to 12 rounds.

Surya Namaskar is not just a physical exercise. For each of the postures, there is a particular breathing pattern to be followed: Inhalation for the backward bends and exhalation for the forwards bends. Further, the concentration has to be focused on a particular *chakra* (energy centre) for each posture, and a particular mantra chanted.

1. **Pranamasana (Prayer Pose):** Stand straight with hands joined together and palms touching each other, near the chest. Keep feet together, heels touching each other and breathe normally.

   Chant*: *Om Mitraaya Namaha (Salutations to the friend of all). Concentrate on the Anahata Chakra (Heart centre).

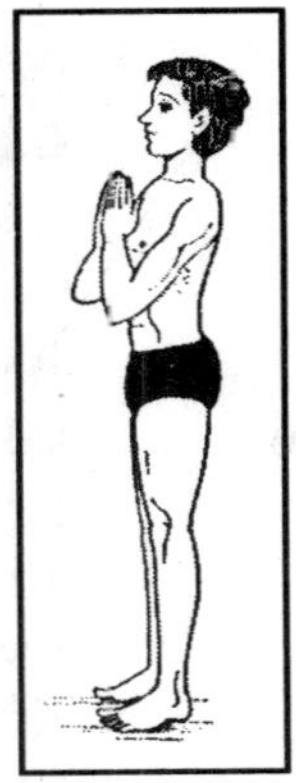

2. **Hasta Uttanasana (Raising Hands):** Inhale, and bend the head backward, looking up. Simultaneously, stretch the hands sideways and up, and join them in the namaskar posture.

   Chant*: *Om Ravaye namaha (Salutation to the Shining One). Concentrate on Vishuddhi Chakra (Throat centre).

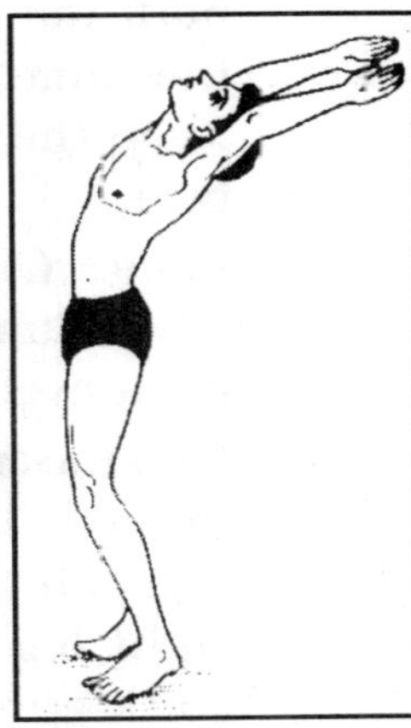

3. **Padahastasana (Toe Touch):** Exhale and bend forward from the waist till palms touch the ground in line with the toes. Don't bend knees while performing. At first you may find it difficult to attain the ideal position but try to

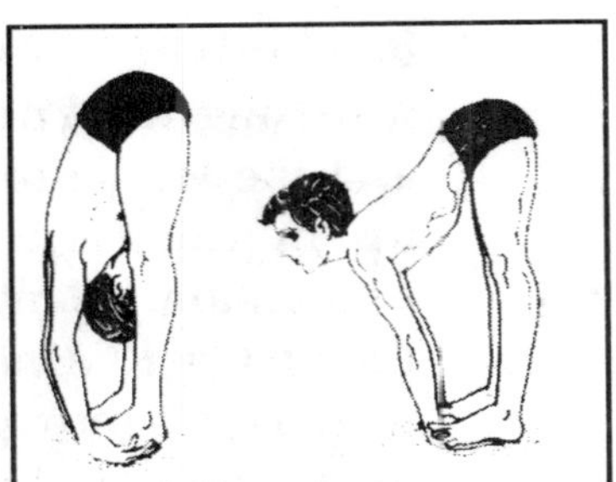

bend as much as possible without bending the knees. ***Chant*: *Om Suryaaya Namaha*** (Salutations to He who induces activity). Focus on Swadishtana Chakra (Sacral centre above the genitals).

4. **Ashwa Sanchalanasana (Horse Pose):** Inhale, and take the left leg back with left toes on the floor, press the waist downward and raise the neck, stretch the chest forward and push the shoulders backward. Keep the right leg and both the hands in the same position. Keep the right leg bent.

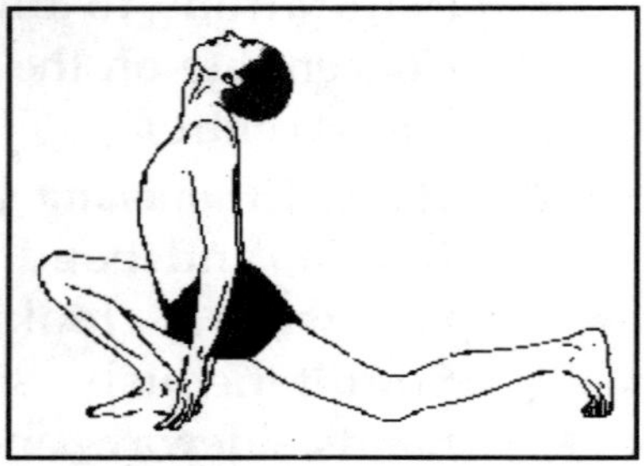

Chant*: *Om Bhaanve Namaha (Salutations to He who illumines). Focus on the Ajna Chakra (Centre of the eyebrows).

5. **Parvatasana (Mountain Pose):** Inhaling, keeping the body balanced on the palms, take the right leg backward and keep it close to the left leg. Let the head be down, eyes watching the knees, and the whole torso up in the form of a mountain, balancing the body on feet and palms.

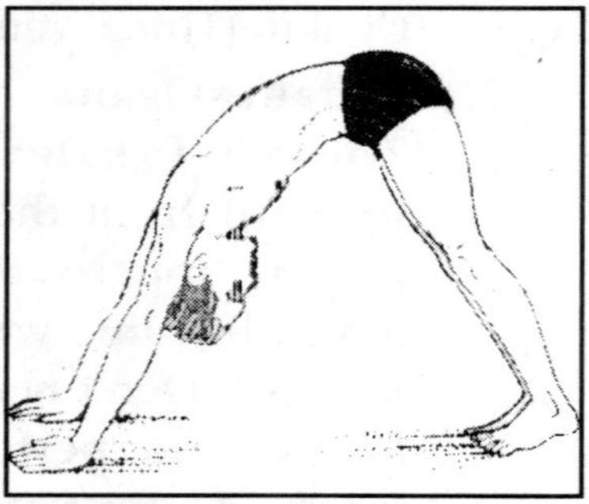

Chant*: *Om Khagaaya Namaha (Salutations to One who moves through the sky). Let the focus be on the Vishuddhi Chakra.

6. **Ashtanga Namaskar (Eight-Limb Salutation):** Exhaling bend both the elbows and touch the forehead on the ground, touch the knees on the ground, keep both the elbows close to the chest. The forehead, chest, both the palms, both the knees and the toes of both feet should touch the ground.

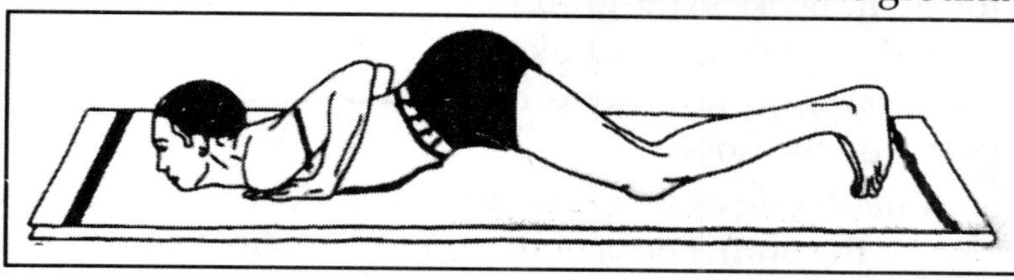

Since only the eight parts rest on the ground, this asana is called 'Ashtanga' pose.

Chant*: *Om Pooshney Namaha (Salutations to the Giver of strength and nourishment). The focus should be on Manipur Chakra (Navel centre).

7. **Bhujangasana (Cobra Pose):** Inhaling straighten the elbows, press the waist downward without bending the arms. Keeping the knees, toes, hips and palms on the floor, bend your head back as far as possible.

Chant*: *Om Hiranyagarbhaya Namaha (Salutations to the Golden Cosmic Self). Focus your attention on Swadishtana Chakra.

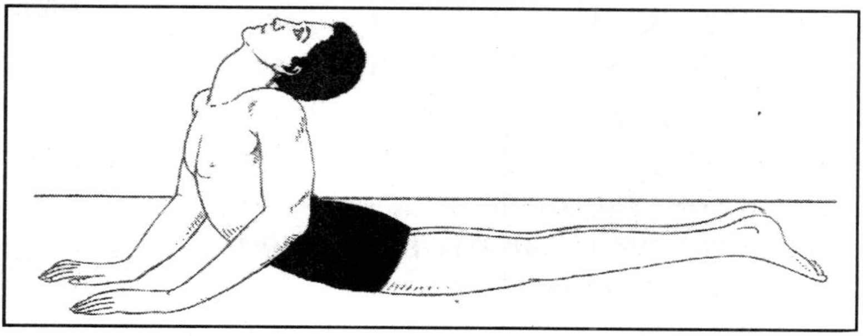

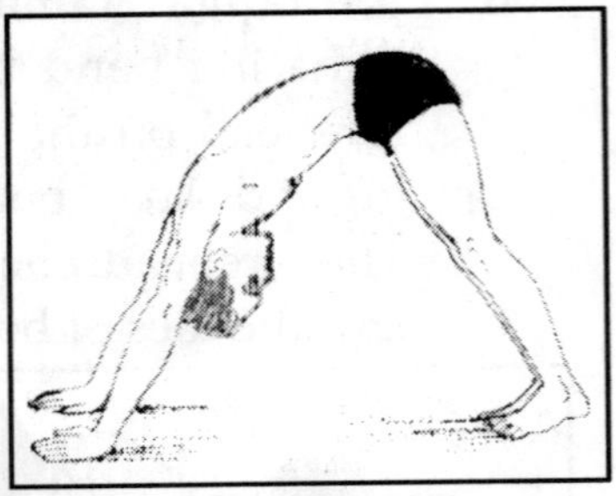

8. Parvatasana (Mountain Pose): Exhaling, bend the neck downward, and press the chin in the throat, push the body backward and touch the heels on the ground, raise the waist upward like a mountain, do not move the palms on the floor.

Chant*: *Om Mareechi-bhyoh Nama (Salutations to the rays of the Sun). Focus your mind on Vishuddhi Chakra.

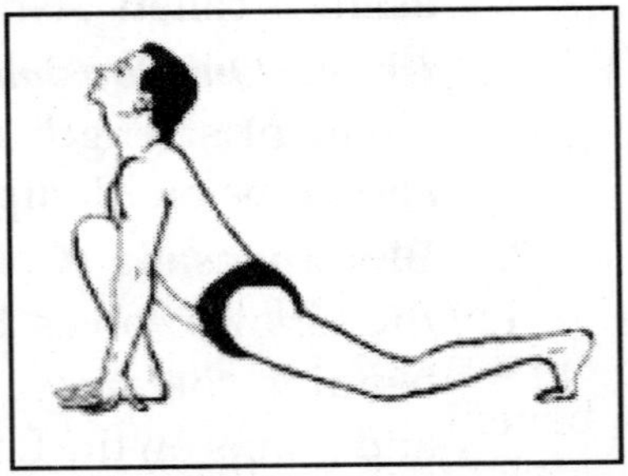

9. Ashwa Sanchalanasana (Horse Pose): Inhaling, bring the right leg in front and place it in between the hands like in position 4, but instead of the left leg in the front here take the right leg, and let the left leg remain at the back with the left knee and toes on the ground.

Chant*: *Om Aadityaaya Namaha (Salutations to the Son of Aditi—the cosmic mother. Focus on Ajna Chakra.

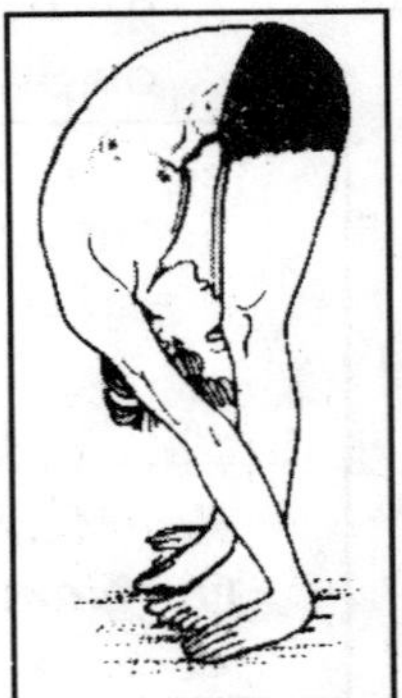

10. Padahastasana (Toe Touch pose): Exhaling, bring the left leg forward near the right leg, between both palms.

Chant*: *Om Savitre Namaha (Salutations to the stimulating power of the Sun). Focus on the Swadishtana Chakra.

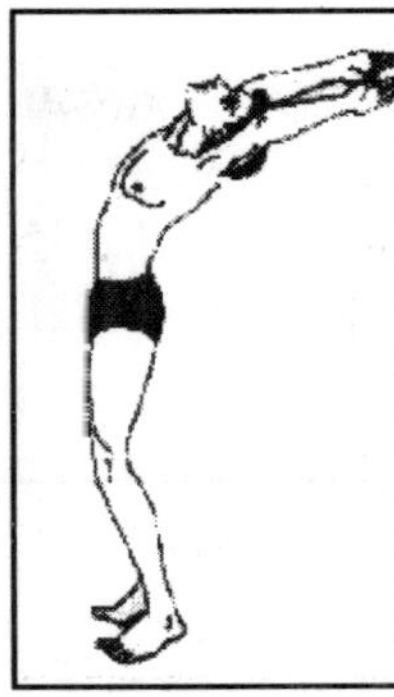

11. Hasta Uttanasana (Arms Lift Pose): Inhaling, raise your body and bending it backward, raise your arms straight up and stretch behind, head up.

Chant: Om Arkaaya Namaha (Salutations to he Who is fit to be praised) Focus on Vishuddhi Chakra.

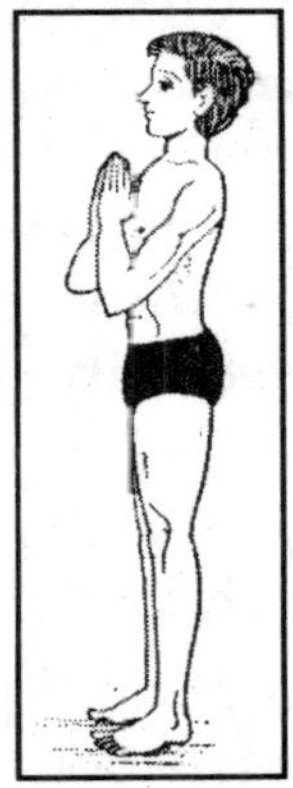

12. Pranamasana (Prayer Pose): Exhaling, bring your hands down to the chest, palms together in the pose of 'namaste', eyes straight ahead, feet together.

Chant: Om Bhaskaraaya Namaha (Salutations to the One Who leads to enlightenment). Focus on Anahata Chakra.

Relax

Surya Namaskar can be done slowly for spiritual benefits and quickly for physical benefits. If doing it quickly, you might find it easier to chant these beeja (seed) mantras for the first six poses:

1. ***Om Hram*** 2. ***Om Hreem*** 3. ***Om Hroom***
4. ***Om Hraim*** 5. ***Om Hraum*** 6. ***Om Hrah***

And then repeat the six mantras again for the next six poses.

Some people chant one mantra per round, and then, at the end of 12 rounds.

Chant

Shree Chhaaya Suvaryalaamba Samet
Shree Surya Narayan Swaminey Namaha
Om Namoh Narayanaaya.

10

PRANAYAMA

A vital scientific and therapeutic aspect of yoga is pranayama. It is the breathing process or the control of the motion of inhalation, exhalation and retention of vital energy. By controlling prana (life force), one can control all the forces of the universe, namely, gravity, magnetism, electricity, and nerve currents.

During pranayama, inhalataion (*punaka*) stimulates the system, and fills the lungs with fresh air; retention (*kumbhaka*) raises the internal temperature and plays an important part in increasing the absorption of oxygen; exhalation (*rechak*) causes the diaphragm to return to the original position, and air full of toxins and impurities is forced out by the contraction of inter-costal muscles. These are the main components of pranayama which massage the abdominal muscles and tone up the working of various organs of the body. Due to the proper functions of these organs, vital energy flows to all the systems. The success of pranayama depends on proper ratios being maintained between inhalation, exhalation and retention.

The lungs are to the body what the bellows are to the fires of the forge. The more regularly and vigorously that the air is forced through the bellows and through the lungs, the livelier burns the flame in the furnace and the fire of life in the body.

Practise deep regular breathing systematically for one week, and you will be surprised at the results. You will feel like a different person, and your working capacity, both physically and mentally, will be increased immensely.

Your breathing is best carried out by lying down on your yoga mat.

'Pranayama' is a compound term (*prana* and *yama*), meaning the maintenance of prana in a healthy state throughout one's life. More than a breath-control exercise, pranayama is all about controlling the life force or prana. Ancient yogis who understood the essence of prana, studied it and devised methods and practices to master it. These practices are better known as pranayama.

Since breath or prana is basic to life, the practice of pranayama helps in harnessing the prana in and around us and by deepening and extending it. Pranayama leads to a state of inner peace. The duration of inhalation, retention and exhalation of breath is regulated with the aim of strengthening and cleansing the nervous system, and increasing a person's source of life energy. There is no doubt that pranayama practice also makes the mind calmer and more focused.

There is no other penance greater than pranayama. It is very important for uprooting the evil thoughts that accumulate over a long time in the mind, and hence refining the mind.

The significance of pranayama is not limited to the quenching of evil customs and purification of mind alone; instead it is related to enhancement of health, mental development, spiritual upliftment and achieving different kinds of spiritual perfection.

Essential Knowledge about Pranayama

In order to practise pranayama fully and effectively, the learner must strictly observe the following rules:

1. **Place:** The place for performing pranayama must be isolated and airy, with ample ventilation.
2. **Time:** The time of dawn is considered as best for practising pranayama. If for any reason it is not possible to practise it in the morning, it can be practised in the evening as well.
3. **Posture:** Mostly the pranayama is practical in Padmasana or Siddhasana. If you face difficulty sitting in these postures for too long, you can select any posture you desire in which you can sit for a long time comfortably.
4. **Bath:** Do not take a bath immediately after Pranayama. You can take it after half an hour of pranayama, though it is better to practise it after a bath, instead of taking a bath after it.

Benefits of Pranayama

Pranayama is like a fire for sin and thus consumes (burns) it, and acts as a bridge to cross the ocean called the world. Asanas destroy the diseases, while sins are destroyed by pranayama. Through pranayama, the spirit of the performance crosses over the barriers, and reaches the brain, and it never dies or falls in the never-ending cycle of birth and death. As a bird tied to a string flies in all the directions but not finding refuge anywhere ultimately returns to its original place, similarly the mind also flies in different directions but ultimately finds support with the soul only because the mind is tied to the spirit. With the circulation of life-giving breath, the mind remains unstable. Dissolving the mind and the spirit in each other, pranayama proves the way for salvation. Hence, pranayama has supreme significance. By regularly performing pranayama, the body remains healthy and free from disease. It also helps in reducing the fat from one's body. It extends your life expectancy, enhances your memory and does away with the mental illness.

Pranayama fully and effectively improves the functioning of the abdomen, liver, urinary track, the intestines and the digestive system. The urine and arteries are purified through pranayama, and physical lethargy is overcome.

Pranayama boosts your appetite and the general health of the body improves. The constant practice of pranayama strengthens the nervous system. The mind becomes calm and capable of concentration, and the spiritual power gets enhanced. The practice of pranayama—the correct breathing technique—helps to manipulate our energies. Most of us breathe incorrectly, using only half of our lung capacity. Pranayama is a technique which re-educates our breathing process, helps us to release tensions and develop a state of mind.

By correctly breathing, your nervous system gets balanced and it encourages creative thinking. According to Patanjali's *Yoga Sutra,* pranayama helps the mind to acquire the capacity to concentrate on any given object of attention. It also says that scientific breathing helps in unveiling true knowledge from the darkness of ignorance. But it is eminently advisable to be aware of the entire do's and dont's of pranayama before practising them. When practised with yogasanas, the benefits of pranayama are more pronounced. With deep breathing exercises, by increasing the amount of oxygen to our brain it improves mental clarity, alertness and physical well-being.

Technique of Pranayama

To practise pranayama, the left and right nostrils are to be closed successively. This is done with the help of the right hand using the right hand thumb. Close the right nostril, and use the ring and little finger of the same hand to close the left nostril. When not using the hands, place them on your knees.

Always inhale and exhale the breath slowly. By doing so the mind remains stable and peaceful. Novices and learners must initially practise inhalation and exhalation; take twice as much time to exhale the breath as they take to inhale. They need to increase the period of breath retention gradually. During the first week, as a beginner, you may retain the breath for four seconds, during the second week for eight seconds, and during the next practice, practice to retain for 12 seconds. Continue the breath up to your full capacity. Don't be discouraged by initial mistakes, and don't drop the practice in panic. You will learn in time. Your common sense, inner wisdom and your soul's voice together tell you the way to perform perfectly.

Various Stages of Pranayama

The following are the stages of pranayama:

1. Inhalation or *puraka*
2. Exhalation of *rechaka*
3. Retention of breath or *kumbhaka*

4. *Ida, pingala and sushumna*
5. Mulabandha, jallundhurbandha and uddiyana-bandha.

It is through various reflex mechanisms that the respiratory system works involuntarily. The depth and rate is maintained automatically according to the oxygen requirements of the body from moment to moment. When the breathing pattern changes during pranayama, the whole mechanism of breathing gets altered. We shall now consider the physiological changes occurring due to the modifications in the breathing pattern during different phases of pranayama.

Puraka

Puraka or inhalation techniques are about regular and controlled inhalation. It also teaches regulating the entire breathing process and reduces the number of inhalations per minute.

The Mechanism of Puraka

Inhalation of air through one or both nostrils.

â

Lungs expand considerably and the walls of the alveoli are stretched to the maximum.

â

Stretch receptors situated in the alveolar walls are stimulated.

â

No exhalation is possible.

â

Chest continues to expand under cortical control.

â

Intra-pulmonary pressure is raised.

â

Diaphragm does not move freely as abdomen is kept slightly inward and controlled.

â

Alveoli in the upper pulmonary are filled with air.

â

The filling of lungs is done as per one's limit and is well intended.

â

A person's inspiratory capacity for prolonged phase of puraka is achieved.

Rechaka

Richaka or exhalation exercises teach slow and ordered breathing besides reducing the number of inhalations and inhalations per minute.

The Mechanism of Rechaka

Exhalation through one nostril or both nostrils.

â

The exhalation is prolonged and the force of going out is reduced.

â

Intra-pulmonary pressure is reduced.

â

The alveoli is greatly deflated.

â

Carbon dioxide increases in the blood.

â

The chemo-receptor tries to inhibit the exhalation and to start the inhalation.

â

Also the peripheral chemo-receptor tries to bring the reflex inspiration.

â

These reflexes help to breathe out.

â

They help to acclimatise the receptors to higher carbon dioxide tension in the blood.

â

As the respiratory reserve volume of the air is used the air containing the carbon dioxide is squeezed out of the lungs.

â

Intra-abdominal pressure is maintained for some time and thus the blood circulation in the lower abdominal regions is diverted towards the sacral region, thus providing nourishment to the parasympathetic branch.

â

A person's capacity for prolonged phase of rechaka is achieved.

Kumbhaka

Kumbhaka consists of retaining the breath after stopping natural inhalation and exhalation. It is about converting both exhalation and inhalation into retention, and storing the retained breath in various internal organs for various lengths of time.

The Mechanism of Kumbhaka

Inhalation is stopped and the inspired air is retained in the lungs for proportionate time.

â

Alveoli and bronchioles are stretched to their optimum level.

â

Stretch receptors, however, cannot string about the reflex contraction of lungs.

â

Respiratory muscles cannot relax as they do normally, due to strong cortical control.

â

Metabolic processes continuously produce carbon dioxide which is picked up by blood.

â

Carbon dioxide concentration increases in blood.

â

Ratio between volumes of inspired air and blood is thus changed.

â

Exchange of oxygen and carbon dioxide, across the thin walls of the alveoli and blood capillaries take place more efficiently.

â

Exchange of gases is not possible after a particular stage when there is a saturation of both gases on both sides—in the alveoli and in blood.

â

Increasing concentration of carbon dioxide in blood stimulates the cranial nerves and chemo-receptors.

â

Sends impulses to respiratory centre.

â

A person is trained to hold his breath.

The Nadis

Kundalini yoga is the yoga of prana. Prana is the life-energy or life-principal of the universe. There are three principal channels through which this life energy flows. These channels are ida, pingala and sushumna. In Sanskrit these channels are called *nadis*. The moon, the sun and the fire are the gods of these nerves or channels, respectively. Ida flows via the left nostril, and pingala flows via the right nostril, while sushumna flows via both the nostrils. Hence sushumna is also called the middle nerve. Ida and pingala keep on changing the tone every hour.

Ida, pingala and sushumna are inside our subtle physical body, not inside the gross physical. Ida carries the current of life-energy in the left side of the body. Pingala carries the current in the right side of the body. Sushumna carries the current in the middle of the spinal column.

Sushumna is the most important of the three *nadis*. It receives a ceaseless stream of life-energy from the universal consciouness—light. There is an inner connection between ida and pingala, and the zodiac and planets. Ida has a special connection with the moon and the planet mercury. Hence its main quality is coolness and mildness. The ida nerve is cool and mainly tamas. It controls the thoughts of the person.

Pingala is connec ed with the sun and Mars, hence its quality is powerful and dynamic heat. Pingala nerve is hot and a mainly rajas in nature. The nerve controls the vital force of life of a person.

Sushumna nerve is also termed as the Brahmanadi. Among all the nerves it is the most important one. It is neither hot nor cool, but maintains a balance between the two. Light and knowledge are gained from this nerve. It helps the learner in spiritual development. From the physical point of view, a balance between these three nerves provides health, vigour, peace and long life.

As stated earlier, ida rules the left nostril while pingala rules the right one. When we breathe in and out primarily through our left nostril. We have to know that it is ida that is functioning. The reverse is the case when pingala is functioning satisfactorily. We have to know that it is sushumna that is playing its role. It also happens at times that ida breathes in and pingala breathes out.

The Bandhas

Bandhas are parts of health-giving poses. During prana-yama, three bandhas are used: Mulabandha, Jallundhar Bandha and Uddiyana Bandha.

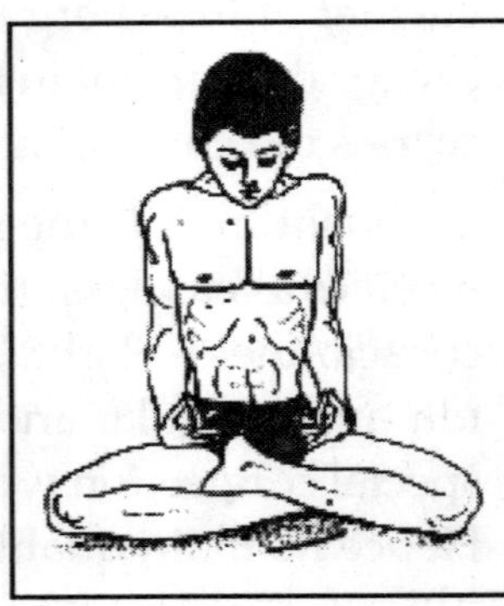

Mulabandha

Press the lower abdominal muscle with the heel of the right foot, and place the heel of the left foot at the base of the genitals. Contracting the arms, pull it forcibly in towards the spinal cord, and feel as if you are trying to pull the wind in your belly. The position of the feet can be interchanged. By practising of pranayama in this bandha or posture you can achieve perfection. Practice of this posture helps one to follow celibacy. This posture stimulates appetite, removes constipation and strengthens virility. It awakens your kundalini. Anyone practising this posture can remain youthful for a longer time.

Jallundhar Bandha

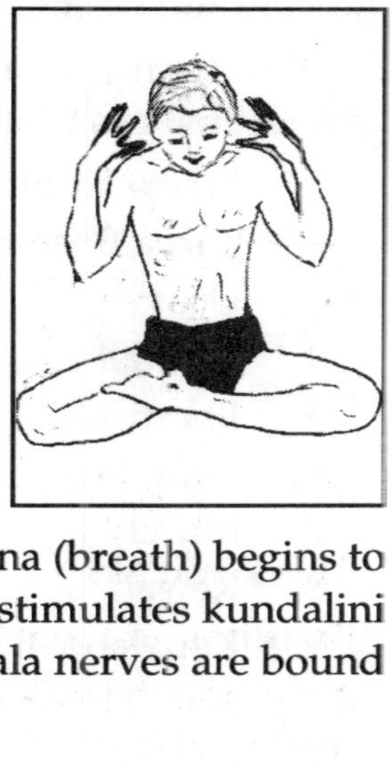

First sit in Padmasana. Contract the throat, and bend the head forward, resting the chin firmly on the chest. The little finger of both hands rest on the shoulders. This bandha is performed at the end of puraka (inhalation) and the beginning of kumbhaka (retention of breath). You must try this bandha only after practising pranayama well.

With practice of this bandha, prana (breath) begins to flow through the prescribed path. It stimulates kundalini power to rise upward. Ida and pingala nerves are bound by the bandha.

Uddiyana Bandha

This method can be practised both in standing and sitting postures. In the standing posture, place your hands on the knees, or on the thighs. Bend your body a little forward while keeping a gap between your feet. Exhaling forcibly, empty your lungs. Contracting the belly, pull the navel and intestines towards your back. Thus you diaphragm will be pushed up as also the wall of the belly. This bandha is practised at the end of kumbhaka and beginning of rechaka.

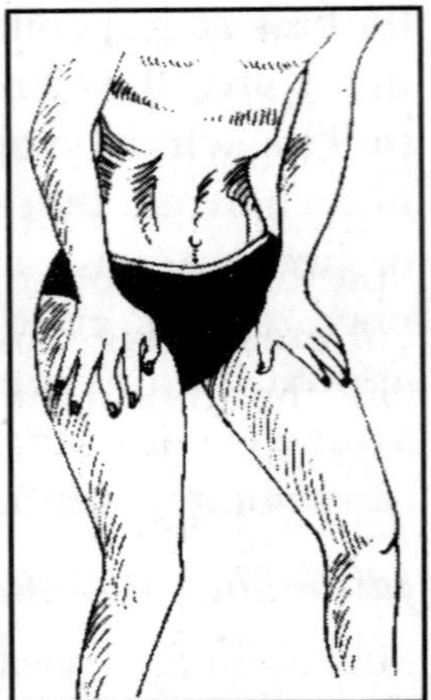

With regular practice of Uddiyana Bandha you may have a youthful look for a very long time. It is extremely helpful in following a celibate life. It awakens the kundalini power, and the body remains healthy and strong.

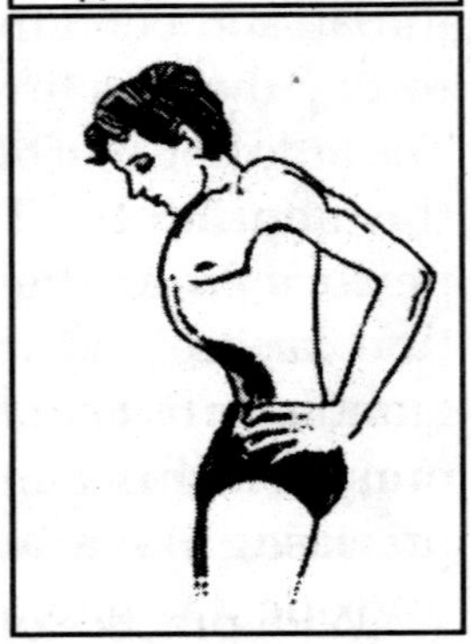

According to Hathayoga, pranayama can be classified under:

1. Sahita Kumbhaka.
2. Surya Bhedan
3. Ujjayi
4. Sheetali
5. Bhastrika
6. Bhramari
7. Murchha
8. Kewali
9. Kapalabhati
10. Nadi Shodhana
11. Agnisar
12. Sheetakari

We will discuss only the important roles.

Kapalabhati

Kapala is Sanskrit word that means 'skull', while *bhati* means 'light' or 'glow'. Thus kapalabhati is a kind of pranayama whose practice makes the skull glow.

Sit down in Padmasana or Siddhasana. Rest your hands on your knees, and close your eyes. Now like the blower of a blacksmith, begin to perform puraka and rechaka (inhalation and exhalation). This exercise must be performed laboriously. There is no kumbhaka or retention of breath stage. Inhalation and exhalation of breath play all the important role. Your nerves will vibrate in this exercise, and you will sweat profusely. It is an extremely powerful exercise performing which all of your cells, neurons and nerves vibrate rapidly.

In the beginning, exhale only once per second. Increase your speed slowly, then exhale twice per second. Initially practise a cycle of 10 exhalations, and then increase the number of exhalations gradually.

Kapalabhati clears your brain, respiratory tract, blood vessels and the sinuses. Destroying the cough that clogs the trachea, kapalabhati leads to the cure of asthma. By constant practice of kapalabhati, air cells in the lungs receive ample amount of life-giving oxygen, hence germs of diseases like tuberculosis cannot harm them. Carbon-dioxide, the gaseous waste of the respiration process, is exhaled out in large amounts, thus purifying the blood. This process also activates the heart and enhances the capacity of the respiratory system, circulation system and digestive system.

Surya Bhedan

Surya bhedan means pricking of the pingala nerve, that is, the nerve of the sun. Thus, the main aim of this pranayama is to awaken the pingala nerve. As a result of this pranayama, that part of the brain which is the abode of masculine power (Shiva) is awakened. The practice of Surya

Bhedan causes a lot of heat to generate in the body. Hence, this pranayama is more beneficial in winters.

Sit in Padmasana or Siddhasana, and close your eyes. Now, close the left nostril with the little finger of your right hand and exhale as deep as you can through your right nostril. Then close the right nostril with the thumb of your right hand and, resting the chin on the chest, retain the breath. Increase the interval of breath retention (kumbhaka) gradually. Then closing your right nostril with the thumb of our right hand, slowly and silently exhale the breath you have so far retained. Repeat the process again.

With regular practice of this pranayama,your mind is refined and the intestinal germs and diseases caused by the wind are destroyed. This pranayama awakens kundalini power as a result of which your appetite is also stimulated. Rheumatic and other wind-causing diseases are corrected. It is excellent to eradicate blood disorders, skin diseases and leprosy. It strengthens the liver, thus helping in the production of bile.

Ujjayi

Since Ujjayi pranayama produces a lot of heat it is best practised in winters.

Sit in Padmasana or Siddhasana. Close your mouth and contract the inner part of the tongue and the wall of throat facing it. Now inhale the breath through both the nostrils and fill your chest with air. Then retain the breath as long as you can do confortably. Ultimately closing the right nostril with the right hand thumb, exhale slowly through the left nostril, expand the chest while you are inhaling the breath. The speed of inhalation must not vary.

With this pranayama, the warmth of the head is reduced, and lung-related diseases like asthma, tuberculosis, etc. are cured. It whets your appetite and enhances the capacity of your digestive system, respiratory system, etc.

Sheetakari

Sheetakari pranayama has a cooling effect on the body and mind.

Sit in Padmasana or Siddhasana. Roll the tongue upward in such a way that its tip touches the upper palate and its mid-part touches the lips. Now suck in the air with an audible s.s.s.s.s... sound. Then retain the breath as long as possible. Ultimately, exhale the breath through both the nostrils. With this practice, hunger, laziness, thirst and excessive sleepiness are eliminated. It prevents over-production of bile. The hardness of the tonsils is also removed. With regular practice of this pranayama, the mental and physical powers of the performer increase.

Sheetali

This too has a cooling effect on the body.

Sit in Padmasana, Siddhasana or Vajrasana. Protruding the tongue, roll it along the sides so that it takes the shape of a blowpipe. Now suck in the air and retain it inside your lungs as long as possible. Finally, exhale the breath slowly through both the nostrils. This type of pranayama expels the toxins

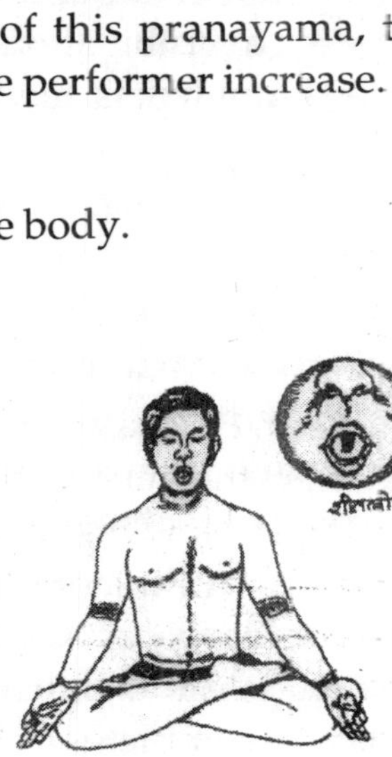

that accumulate in the blood, and thus purifies the blood. Diseases like tumour, jaundice, skin eruptions, and fever are cured, and it corrects indigestion and constipation. It quenches the thirst also. Hence, if for any reason, getting drinking water is not possible at some place and you are very thirsty, you may quench the thirst through this pranayama.

With regular practice of this, you may become immune to snakebite and scorpion stings. For the short-tempered people and those who get excited quickly, this pranayama is highly beneficial. It also helps in toning up the liver and spleen, and leprosy or gangrene can be prevented.

Bhastrika

Bhastrika means bellows. Hence exhalation of breath forcible and quickly is the main feature of this pranayama. One should inhale and exhale like a blower or bellow. It is, in a way, a combination of Kapalabhati and Ujjayi. Among all the kumbhakas, this pranayama is considered to be the best.

Sit in Padmasana or Siddhasana. Stretch your head, neck and back. Place your hands on your lap or knees. Inhale and exhale rapidly four or five times like the bellows. Similarly, contract and expand the lungs. A peculiar rolling sound will be produced during the practice of this pranayama. But you must perform this rapidly and without stopping even once.

At the completion of one cycle (*avartana*) inhale the breath as deeply as possible, and retain it as long as possible. Finally, exhale as much breath as possible. Thus a cycle of bhastrika completes.

After resting for a while, perform another cycle of this

pranayama. Perform three cycles of this each day. Initially, you can start with a single cycle, gradually building it up to three cycles. Perform this pranayama twice—once in the morning and once in the evening—in winters, and only once a day in summers.

With the practice of Bhastrika, the swelling in the throat is removed, your cough gets cured and your appetite gets whetted. Diseases of the nose and chest, like asthma, sinusitis, etc. are cured. Ailments caused by imbalance of wind, cough and bile are corrected. The pores of the sushumna nerve are opened by Bhastrika.

Bhramari

This term originates from the Sanskrit word *Bharmar*, meaning 'bumblebee'. While performing this pranayama, a buzzing sound, typical of a bumblebee, is produced from the nostrils.

Sit down in Padmasana or Siddhasana. Inhale and exhale breaths rapidly through both the nostrils with a buzzing sound like that of a bumblebee. Continue doing this till you sweat profusely. End this exercise with inhalation of the breath through the nostrils as deeply as possible, and hold it as long as you can. Then exhale through both the nostrils. As you increase the speed of inhalation and exhalation of breath, the blood circulation improves, leading to generation of heat in the body, and profuse sweating. This sweating cools down your body and you will experience a joyful sensation.

With this pranayama, your mood gets elevated with joy, with increased flow of knowledge and asceticism sets in. With successful practice of kumbhaka, the performer enters successfully into a stage of trance or samadhi.

Murchha

Murchha means 'unconsciousness'. Through this pranayama the performer attains Murchhavastha, or the state of unconsciousness or coma, and his mind becomes free of all feelings.

Sit down comfortably in a posture that best suits you. Inhale the breath through both the nostrils deeply. Then retain the breath with the help of a powerful Jullundhar Bandha. Finally, exhale the breath through both the nostrils. The mind becomes free of all feelings and you experience elation and joy. Thoughts and resolutions decrease in the mind, and you experience the feeling of non-existence, that is, the *mana* (mind) becomes *amana* (mindless), and merges in ethereal energy cell Paramatma.

Plavini

This term originated from the Sanskrit word *plu* meaning 'to float'; thus, plavini means the one that causes to float.

Initially, practise this pranayama in Siddhasana or Vajrasana. With practice you can perform it in standing or lying posture as well. If you are performing it in a sitting posture, inhale the breath through both the nostrils and retain it by Jallundhar Bandha. When you take Jallundhar Bandha, the retained air fills the intestines which get inflated as a result. End the pranayama with exhalation of breath through both the nostrils. If necessary, remove the air that is trapped in the intestines by Uddiyana Bandha.

A person who is a master of this art of pranayama can sustain his life for many days without food. During its practice, the blood flows in the body extremely fast, thus removing the impurities and toxins accumulated in the body. With the practice of this pranayama, the performer gains the power to float on water. An expert can even remain floating on deluging waters like a light lotus leaf. For the perfection of this pranayama, slow but continuous and regular practice is extremely essential.

Pancha Prana

Five subtle streams, called Pancha Prana, of *Prana Shakti* flow in a human being. These are described in the Indian scriptures as five divine powers (*Pancha Deva*) manifested in the human body. The extrasensory scriptures serpentine power centre (*Kundalini*) is said to be subtly containing an unlimited repository of prana shakti. The higher level endeavours of prana yoga attempt stimulation, stirring, upthrust and elevation of the flow of prana. The power of prana in a human being is divided into 10 categories according to its manifestation in different regulatory and vital activities. Five major types, called pancha prana, under this classification are:

1. Apana
2. Samana
3. Prana
4. Udana
5. Vyana

The five subtypes, or upa pranas, are:

1. Devadatta
2. Vrakala
3. Koorma
4. Napa
5. Dhananjaya

Each stream of the five major pranas activate specific

physiological and bodily process, and is also associated with the extrasensory centres (ESC) governing the endocrine system.

1. ***Apana***
   Regulates excretion of waste and obnoxious substances from the body, it is linked with the Mooladhara chakra (the root centre or ESC in the pelvic plexus).
2. ***Samana***
   Activates the metabolic process and is regarded as the source of power in the Manipuraka chakra (solar plexus or ESC in the epigastric plexus).
3. ***Prana***
   It is the source of respiration and is associated with the Anahata chakra (heart centre or ESC in the cardiac plexus).
4. ***Udana***
   Regulates the processes of acceptance and absorption of desired elements in the body, and also used in upward motion. It is the source of activation in the Vishuddhi chakra (throat centre, or ESC in the carotid plexus).
5. ***Vyana***
   Regulates blood circulation, and is described as the source of power for the Swadhisthana chakra (sacral centre just above the genitals, or ESC in hypogmistric plexus).

❑❑❑

11

MEDITATION

In today's world, most popular are worried and stressed over finances, emotional family situations, relationship and sickness. This produced stress and emotional reactions that can lead to illness on several levels. Our bodies and minds can tolerate only so much of any of these. After a while, each of us reaches a saturation point, and the results become uncomfortable at best; for some it may be unbearable even unendurable.

While there is no guaranteed cure to eliminate stress and anxiety there is a solution that helps to balance the mental, emotional, physical and spiritual state of well-being. The answer is inside of all of us. We must go inside ourselves. This process is known as meditation. You may want to view your time learning to meditate as time spent for yourself. Giving yourself attention is a must since most of the time is spent worrying about others and how to take care of those around us.

This is a self-care activity: loving yourself! The peace and joy felt by those who meditate is invaluable. This practice can be used to facilitate healing.

An ordinary person may consider meditation as a worship or prayer. But it is not so. Meditation means awareness. Whatever you do with awareness is meditation. 'Watching our breathe, is meditation; listening to the birds is meditation. As long as these activities are free from any other destruction to the mind, it is effective meditation. Meditation is not a technique but a way of life. Meditation means 'to join together or to yoke'. It describes a state of consciousness, when the mind is free of scattered thoughts and various patterns. The observer (one who is doing meditation) realises that all the activity of the mind is reduced to one.

These days it is commonly understood to mean some form of spiritual practice where one sits down with eyes closed, and empties the mind to attain inner peace, relaxation or even an experience of God. The word 'meditation' is derived from two Latin words: *meditare* (to think, to dwell upon, to exercise the mind) and *mederi* (to heal). Its Sanskrit derivation *medha* means wisdom.

Many years ago, meditation was considered something just not meant for modern people with all types of people. Published scientific and medical evidence has proved its benefits, but it still needs to be understood. Traditionally, the classical yoga texts describe that, to attain true states of meditation, one must go through several stages. After the necessary preparation of personal and social code, physical position, breath control and relaxation come the more advanced stages of concentration, contemplation and then, ultimately absorption. But that does not mean that one must perfect any one stage before moving onto the next. The integral yoga approach is simultaneous application of a little of all stages together.

Commonly today, people can mean any one of the these stages when they refer to the term 'meditation'. Some schools only teach concentration techniques, some relaxation, and others teach free contemplative activities like just sitting and awaiting absorption. Some call it meditation without giving credence to yoga for fear of being branded 'eastern'. But yoga is not something eastern or western, as it is universal in its approach and application. With regular practice of a balanced series of techniques, the energy of the body and mind can be liberated, and the quality of consciousness can be expanded. This is not a subjective claim, but it now being investigated by the scientists, and being shown by an empirical fact. Meditation is one of the five principles of yoga. It is the practice by which there is constant observation of the mind. It requires you to focus your mind at one point, and still the mind in order to perceïve the self. Through the practice of meditation you will achieve a greater sense of purpose and strength of will. It also helps you achieve a clearer mind, improve your concentration, and discover the wisdom and tranquillity within you.

Meditation is also one of the eight limbs of yoga which leads to samadhi or enlightenment. Research shows that the practice of meditation contributes to our physical and psychological well-being. It can reduce blood pressure, and relieve stress and pain. Meditating also brings our mind to a level of consciousness that promotes healing or what is known as the alpha state. Achieving the alpha state can help decrease anxiety, depression and other mental, psychological or emotional problems.

In yoga meditation, we learn to train the being to tune itself to the working of the Divine Being. The Central principle of such meditation is to concentrate one's mental faculties upon the object of quest. But this requires long hours of practice for the mind to be able to attain such sustainable levels of concentration and absorption. This discipline, above everything else, is the essence of yoga meditation. The success of yogic meditation depends largely on the sincerity and strength of yogi behind it. It is not the duration but the intensity of the aspiring consciousness which is more important and ultimately effective. Fatigue is to be avoided at all costs since it weakens the power of concentration and jades the mind. Yoga meditation puts the being of the meditating yogi in a condition of increased and conscious receptivity to the working of yoga shakti or the power of yoga. With a deepening of this state of mind there is often a total withdrawal from the eternal environment.

Through meditation we temporarily withdraw ourselves from the many superficial activities of the day, and turn our attention inward. In doing so, we gradually come to perceive the source of our existence, and automatically integrate ourselves with this source. We allow ourselves more and more, to become expressions, sounding boards as it were, of the Absolute, of God. As this begins to occur, the individual is freed from the terribly confining limitations of what he has heretofore conceived of as 'me' or 'I', and the necessity of protecting the phantom known as the 'ego'. The implications of this cannot be overstated. Energies released from the carrying of the ego burden are tremendous, and affect, in an undesirable manner, every aspect of our lives. The consciousness is greatly elevated, and the resulting state of existence can only be hinted at with words such as 'joy', 'bliss' and 'true peace'.

Method of Yoga Meditation

The following are a few tips to remember while practising yoga meditation.

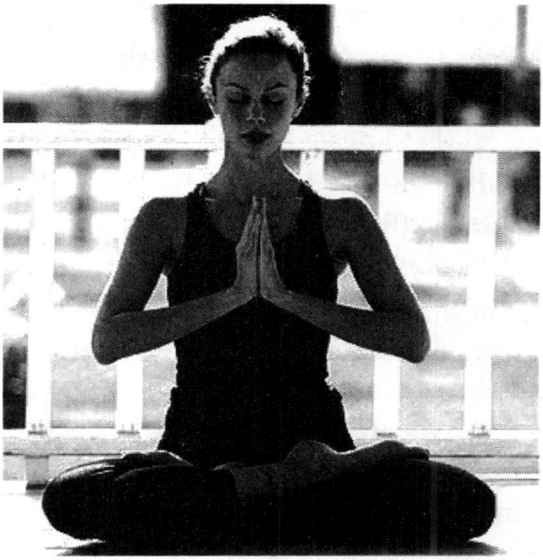

1. Meditation can be practised whenever you feel the need for renewal, or following yogasanas.
2. Sit in a comfortable posture with an erect spine, preferably in a specific yogasana such as Padmasana or Siddhasana. The Padmasana postures are the result of painstaking experiments by the great yogis of the past to perfect a position in which frequent movement of the legs would not be required (as the body moves, the mind is distracted). This asana also enables the spine to be erect and the body firmly rooted.
3. Assume the anjali mudra pose at first (anjali mudra explained below).
4. Then the eyelids are lowered, not closed.
5. The tips of the forefinger and thumbs are joined to form a circle, while the other fingers are extended.
6. Breathing will be slowed automatically.

7. Energise the breath through pranayama.
8. Hold a visualisation for a few minutes to clear the sensory field, and focus the mind internally. This may relate to peaceful colours, geometric designs, natural images or that of a deity or guru.
9. Repeat an affirmation or chant or prayer to increase positive power.
10. Repeat a mantra such as 'Om' to still the mind. Ideally, one should repeat a mantra at least 108 times before meditation.
11. Having resolved, gently but firmly, not to be distracted, you remain motionless in this position for as long as is comfortable, becoming acutely aware of what is occurring within.
12. As you silently observe the mind, let it empty it self out.
13. Depending on your natural temperament, it would help to try and establish contact with either God or a higher consciousness through the natural movement of your heart.

Anjali Mudra

Anjali means 'offering', and in India, this mudra is often accompanied by the word 'namaste'. If you have attended even one yoga class, it is a familiar gesture: the drawing together of one's palms at the heart. Your teacher may bring his or her hands together while saying 'namaste' at the beginning or end of a class. You may find this gesture with certain asanas, as in Tadasana (Mountain Pose), before you begin Surya Namaskar, or in balance pose such as Vrukshasana (Tree Pose). This sacred hand position, called anjali mudra, is found throughout Asia, and has become synonymous with images of the east, from the smiling face of the Dalai Lama peering over his fingertips of images of devotees before a Hindu or Buddhist altar. In the west, this gesture is translated as a posture of prayer. Since we have grown up with this posture as part of our culture, each of us probably has his own personal connection to this mudra—positive or negative. Some of us may find a subconscious resistance to bringing our hands together as if it were a sign of submission. However, the beauty of this gesture, which positions us right at the of core our being, us timeless and universal.

As we explore the significance and potential of this mudra, be open to your own experience and ways that this simple yet powerful hand position can be a practical tool in your practice and daily life. In Sanskrit, *mudra* means 'seal' or 'sign', and refers not only to sacred hand gestures but also whole body positions that elicit a certain inner state or symbolise a particular meaning.

Anjali mudra is but one of thousands of types of mudras that are used in Hindu rituals, classical dance and yoga. As the consummate Indian greeting, like a sacred hello, this mudra is often translated as, "I bow to the Divinity within you from the Divinity within me". This salutation is at the essence of the yogic practice of seeing the Divine within all of creation. Hence, this gesture is offered equally to temple deities, teachers, elders, strangers, and before sacred rivers and trees. Anjali mudra is used as a posture of composure, of returning to one's heart, whether you are greeting someone, or saying goodbye, initiating or completing an action. As you bring your hands together at the centre, you are literally connecting the right and left hemispheres of your brain. This is the yogic process of unification, the yoking of our active and receptive natures. In the yogic view of the body, the energetic or spiritual heart is visualised as a lotus at the centre of the chest. Anjali mudra nourishes this lotus heart with awareness, gently encouraging it to open, as water and light do a flower.

Bowing the head and closing the eyes, with hands in anjali mudra help the mind surrender to the Divine in the heart. One can do namaste to oneself as a meditation technique to go deeper inside the heart chakra; when done with someone else, it is also a beautiful, albeit quick, meditation. For a teacher and student, namaste allows two individuals to come together energetically to a place of connection and timelessness, free from the bonds of ego connection. If it is done with deep feeling in the heart and with the mind surrendered, a deep union of spirits can blossom. The teacher initiates anjali mudra as a symbol of gratitude and respect towards her students and her own teachers, and in return invites the students to connect with their lineage, thereby allowing the truth to flow—the truth that we are all one when we live from the heart.

Some Common Chants

The following are some chants commonly used that are helpful at the start of meditation.

1. *Aum*

   The primal *shabda* or sound that is actually pronounced 'Aum' and not 'Om', it is an affirmation of the Divine Presence that is the universe, and is similar to the Hebrew 'Amen'. There are many ways of chanting *Aum*, but this is an approach that will initiate you as a true yogi, one who pursues the path of sound toward wholeness and higher states of consciousness.

2. ***Lokah Samastha***

   A chant for wholeness, *Lokah samastha sukhino bhavantu* (May this world be established with a sense of well-being and happiness).

3. ***Gayatri***

   Being illuminated by Sacred Sound. *Om bhur bhuvas svaha, that savithur varaynyam, bhargo devasya dhimahih, dhiyo yonah pratchodhayat.* (We worship the word—*shabda*—that is present in the earth, the heavens, and that which is beyond. By meditating on this glorious power that gives us life, we ask that our minds and hearts be illuminated).

4. *Om Namah Shivaaya, Om Namah Shivaaya, Namah Shivaaya, Nama Shiva* (I bow to Lord Shiva, the peaceful One Who is the embodiment of all that is caused by the universe).

❑❑❑

12

WEIGHT REGULATION

If you have ever tried to lose weight, then you probably already know that doctors and weight loss diets and programmes only bring temporary reliefs or results.

Each person who is overweight has an individual problem, since his metabolism and certain other vital factors are different from those of his neighbour. Due to these differences, the amount of food that constitutes 'overeating' and the amount of activity that constitutes 'adequate exercise', vary with the individual. Among your friends you can observe those who eat heavily at meal time, pack in several between-meal snacks and perhaps do very little active work or exercising during the day, and yet may be less overweight than yourself or others who are watching their diets carefully and are quite active. What accounts for this apparent discrepancy? The simple fact is: bodies function differently with regard to metabolic process.

If you take some diet pills, you may lose weight because your appetite is temporarily suppressed. When you stop taking the pills your appetite will return and you will be faced with the same problem. The pills are a short-term solution, and in some cases may even be harmful to you. If you adopt an extreme weight loss diet you may get dramatic results while you stay on the diet, but if you live a normal life, surrounded by your family and friends, you probably will not be able to stay on that diet for a long time. As soon as you quit the diet and return to your old ways, you will gain weight again. In addition, as with pills, many weight loss diets are not healthy, and can even be harmful.

For a long-term weight loss you need to go to the root of the problem, and value changes in your life and lifestyle. Excess weight in our society is mostly due to a sedentary lifestyle and poor selection of food. It may also be due to psychological stress, and in some cases metabolic problems (that is, your body is not efficient in turning food into energy). Yoga provides a powerful alternative to conventional weight loss programmes and plans, and is helpful in combating all the causes of obesity and excess weight accumulation. Why? Because yoga is not a conventional sport or exercise. Yoga is system of personal transformation on all levels—physical, mental and spiritual.

You go to a lecture on nutrition and they tell you that eating too many fatty foods will lead to obesity. After you attend the lecture your know that it is not healthy to eat a lot of junk food. But when you get on the street and go past a fast food restaurant you get hungry. Intellectually you know that it is not good to eat junk food, but can you control yourself? Sadly, the answer is usually no.

Our body is like a chariot pulled by horses. The horses are our desires and the various organs that they use to fulfil themselves such as hands, feet, mouth, etc. Sometimes these desires are running like horses out of control. Our mind knows so many things and wants to chart a sensible path, but our mind is not strong enough to reign in the wild horses. Yoga helps you to put your mind in control. It helps you to have the strength to do the right thing at the right time. Yoga will show you how to do physical exercises and meditation exercises that will gradually change you from the inside out. It is good if you can stop or check a desire to do the wrong thing; it is even better if this desire never arises in your mind. The effects of yoga are to make deep-rooted changes in your inner being. As you feel more relaxed and calm, nervous eating will vanish.

Since no two people are alike, the necessity of learning to truly 'know thyself' can be appreciated. 'Knowing' yourself entails turning away more and more from those outside sources that want to tell you how you should look, what you should weigh, how to make yourself beautiful, and so on, and, in place of these, undertaking a perceptive self-examination, for example, you must no longer ampute your correct weight from the charts on the scales of those listed in books and magazines, for all people cannot have identical bone structures.

Rather, you should learn to know at what weight you are functioning at your best; and in a similar vein, exactly how the foods you are eating affect you, as well as the values that various sports exercise routines and other activities hold for you. If a large-boned woman attempts to model her measurement after those of the mannequins in the fashion magazines, she will not only be frustrated in her attempt but she can actually find herself in serious physical trouble. She simply is not meant by nature to resemble a mannequin. However, if this same woman will proportion her weight correctly, improve her muscle tone, make her skin taut and firm, develop an erect posture and move with poise and balance, she will reveal herself as confident, vital and harmonious as was nature's intention. Each woman is beautiful in her own right.

If you learn how to apply yoga to your life, you will get a long-term solution to the problem to achieving self-control and self-fulfilment. Without any special equipment you will be able to do exercises that keep you in shape; you will learn how to do meditation that will put your mind at peace; you will become internally balanced, and you will make the choices that are right for you. Why wait any longer? You can read hundreds of web pages or books about weight reduction or weight loss, but if you only read and don't practise, you are not going to go anywhere.

If you can find time for half an hour of exercises in the morning and half an hour in the evening, then you can do it. You don't need super will power and self-discipline to do it; you will actually acquire greater will power and self-discipline by practising the exercises to the best of your capacity. You don't need athletic ability or a flexible body; if you can even try to stretch, you will get the full benefits of yoga.

In yoga, there is a unique and wonderfully natural approach to weight regulation. The postures are performed without strain and with minimum effort, and are designed to stimulate and promote the correct functioning of the important organs and glands that are weight-control factors, and that receive so little conscious attention in the usual systems of exercising or in the use of 'reducing' machines.

Specially, you will be working on the thyroid gland, improving blood circulation, breathing in a way designed to burn excess fat and strengthening many areas where you will find that weight is more easily removed when they are firmed. Each yoga exercise will, in one way or another, aid you in weight regulation and control. Even those stretching and breathing techniques designed to alleviate tension are helpful since the desire of the compulsive eater can often be diminished if nervous disturbances are reduced.

It is a basic concept of yoga, with regard to the problem of weight regulation, that the wisdom and intelligence of your own body are much greater than all of the 'miracle diets', the ingenious exercising machines and devices, the calorie-counting charts and various reducing gimmicks. If you will learn to listen to what your body is really telling you, you can accomplish many of your physical objectives, including those of weight regulation and control.

As the life-force is increased through your yoga practice, the intelligence and wisdom that lie within you will make you actually aware of those things that are of benefit to your organism and those that are harmful.

The phrase 'weight control' may be ill-chosen. 'Control' usually implies a battle. When you undertake a programme of 'control' you are prepared for restrictions and denials and this places you at a psychological disadvantage. Since you will have such strong, positive mind in normalising your weight through yoga, it is better to speak here in terms of 'weight regulation'. You select the foods you know your body requires rather than deny yourself what your taste buds and eyes desire. You practise your yoga exercise because they are enjoyable and rewarding, rather than forcing yourself to huff and puff away a few pounds as is the case in most other methods of exercising.

If you do the simple exercises on a daily basis, then in a period of three to six months you will begin to feel and see changes in yourself, and in one year's time you will be able to enjoy your new 'look, and better health.

Remember, regular yoga practice can help in weight regulation. Firstly, some of asanas stimulate the sluggish glands to increase their hormonal secretions. The thyroid gland, especially, has a big effect on your weight because it affects body metabolism. There are several asanas, such as Sarvangasana and Matsyasana which are specific for the thyroid gland. Fat metabolism is also increased, so fat is converted to muscle and energy. This means that, as well as losing fat, you will have better muscle tone, and a higher vitality level. The following asanas and programme are beneficial in weight loss:

1. **Surya Namaskar**

   This is a composite exercise that includes different asanas. It strengthens and activates sluggish stomach, lungs, liver, spleen, intestines and spinal cord. The entire body, especially the waist, gains the elasticity and fat gets reducesd.

2. **Naukasana (Boat Pose)**

   This tones up the digestive system, and fights obesity.

3. **Supta Vajrasana**

   The fat from knees, thighs, waist, abdomen, neck and ankles melt down. The muscles in them get strengthened.

4. **Mayurasana**

   Besides checking obesity, it enhances the functioning of the kidneys and digestive organs, removing all problems related to wind, bile and phlegm. It increases blood circulation in the body and purifies the blood. It also removes sluggishness from the liver.

5. **Paschimottanasana**

   Obesity, piles, backache and constipation all disappear with the regular practice of this asana. It helps to strengthen the sushumna nadi, and increases the elasticity of the spine, thereby giving perennial youth. Disorders of the kidney, liver and spleen are removed.

6. **Makarasana**

   This has a particularly good effect on reducing the flab from the abdomen. The back and neck become resilient, and blood circulation increases.

7. **Halasana**

   While strengthening the pancreas, spleen, liver and kidneys, this asana is very effective in reducing obesity, especially from the waist and abdomen.

Pranayama too is very beneficial in weight regulation.

❑❑❑

13

YOGA DIET

Yoga is the only science that has laid great emphasis on food over centuries. In fact, there is a whole branch, called Anna Yoga, devoted to food for health and happiness.

Yoga over centuries has developed a concept of a balanced whole-food diet and an eating philosophy. These principles of good eating use powerful techniques which help in maintaining a strong and healthy body, a stress-free mind and a positive spiritually within this mixed-up world.

Never has this yogic philosophy of a balanced whole-food diet been felt more than today when 97 per cent of all health disorders can be traced to a faulty nutrition and diet.

The chief sources of life-force are air, water, sleep, food and sunlight. Breathing, drinking and sleeping are almost automatic processes about which there is not too much choice. You must continually breathe; you drink when you are thirsty, and generally sleep when tired. But you are free to choose from a multitude of food products. Therefore, it is essential that the yoga student understand certain vital principles regarding this choice.

You must make certain that you are getting the most possible life-force from the foods that you eat. Otherwise, since foods can sap your vitality as well as nourish you, your eating habits may well be doing you more harm than good! By eating too often and consuming too many heavy, rich, indigestible and devitalised foods you will allow your stomach to drain vital energies from other parts of your body, especially from your physical defence agents and your mental and spiritual bodies. The yogi believes that the less you eat, the better you will feel, providing your food is of high quality.

If you are forcing your body to digest several of the typical junk meals each day, you may well find that your strength, vitality and endurance are decreased, and that your mind functions less efficiently.

Your organism is a precision instrument designed to function at its peak on small amounts of high-quality food. Such light, high quality food, eaten sparingly, has the ability to nourish you and leave important vital energies free to help activate those little-used forces with which we are concerned.

Overeating as well as incorrect eating may also be the cause of a great many physical disorders. Indeed, certain nutritionists believe that almost all illnesses can be attributed directly or indirectly to the toxins, acids and waste products continually formed by inferior foods that cannot be properly digested and eliminated. These nutritionists maintain that the body is capable of coping with most germs that enter it, providing that this body is in a pure, clean, healthy state with the ability to call upon its defence agents as needed. But a physical organism that is low in resistance because its defence agents are occupied in other areas, trying to cope with toxins, congestions and deposits, is greatly weakened in its attempt to fight these germs. Therefore, the yoga student must make certain that her diet does not inhibit either the life-force already existent in the organism or the new life-force that will be gained through the yoga exercises.

It has been observed that Indians suffer least from bowel problems, constipation, indigestion and other food-related disorders such as obesity. This is because the Indian philosophies of cooking and eating draws heavily from the yogic philosophy of eating.

Yoga does not dissect food into vitamins, minerals, proteins, etc. The yogic philosophy is that the true benefits of these ingredients can be had only when they are not isolated but as much in their natural form as possible.

All foods should be consumed in a form that is as close to the natural state as digestion permits. In their natural state, most foods contain life-force. When foods are boiled, fried, roasted, refined, canned, frozen, preserved, fumigated, aged, pasteurised, 'enriched' and otherwise subjected to the innumerable modern processes, the life-force is seriously reduced or killed. You can fill your stomach and appear to satisfy your hunger with boiled vegetables, frozen fruits, aged cheeses, white bread, refined sugar candies, etc., but the real nourishment, or life-force, of these products is highly questionable. Thus the yogi is concerned not with the amount of food he eats but with the amount of life-force in that food.

It is said that our level of development—mental and spiritual—is reflected in the kind of food we eat, and our stage of consciousness is revealed in the nature of that chosen food. Both yoga and ayurveda advise on a sattvic or a pure vegetarian diet. Such a diet, it is believed, encourages the development of the higher qualities of peace, love and spiritual awareness.

The basis of an ideal sattvic diet is the attitude of ahimsa or non-violence. A sattvic or ascetic diet is first and foremost purely vegetarian, eschewing all such methods which involve the killing of animals. In addition, a lot of emphasis is put on natural foods, that is, foods grown in harmony with nature, on good soils, ripened naturally, cooked in the right manner and with the right attitude of love. Partaking of diet such as this helps in the development of prana or vital energy and spiritual consciousness.

Yogic diet is best suited not only for detoxification of the body but also for burdening the parameters of our mind. And for the same reason, die-hard yogis recommend raw foods coupled with frequent fruits. They believe that a reduction in a body ultimately results in the expansion and development of the mind-increasing detachment, and lowering our physical consciousness while raising the spiritual counterpart.

Food is central to good health. It is medicine you take every day and so is the most important factor in maintaining good health and in avoiding disease. In the process of trying to establish good eating habits, it is not necessary or even desirable to become food obsessed, that is, weighing, measuring, analysing your food, rather if you adhere to a general principle of right eating you can achieve much more stable results. Eating fresh whole natural foods, in balanced proportions, is the only diet that most of you will ever need to follow.

There are several reasons that the body needs to desire food. One is to supply it with energy so that it can continue its normal functioning. The body also needs food to repair tissues and organs, these are the two primary reasons for eating food, but since the body is subservient to the mind, the mind also creates reasons to eat. For instance, food is often used as a substitute for love and affection, or as a means to relieve tension or fear, or it may also be used to relieve bordom or depression. These are not good reasons to eat, and so all these psychological factors must be dealt with before a good diet can have any lasting effect.

Before focusing on what specific foods are recommended by the philosophy of yoga, it is important to discuss the relationship between overeating and ill-health. It is essential for you to learn to control your consumption of food. By controlling the amount of food your consume, and this is regardless of what kinds of foods you may be consuming, you can contribute significantly to a long and healthy life. Overeating is one of the causes of diseases and early death. It has been proved in study after study of the most long-lived people of the world that the most common denominator in each individuals lifestyles is the fact that they all eat very sparingly.

The key to true health is to have a balanced whole-food diet. A balanced diet ensures that all the faculties of digestion work smoothly—absorption, assimilation and elimination. A balanced whole-food diet ensures a healthy you!

It is extremely important that all these three aspects work well together. If all these aspects work in harmony it is extremely unlikely that you'll suffer from health disorders and even obesity. Often 'synthetic' or 'processed' foods create conditions that disrupt this balance. This leads to several physical and psychological problems. Over years, this can have dangerous consequences.

So what are whole-foods? They are edible substances which are as close to their 'whole' or natural state as possible. They have not been pre-processed in anyway which would disturb their nutrition or flavour. They are therefore free of all processing additives or subtractions.

The overall idea of whole-foods is to buy foods which are:

1. As whole and in their most simple form as possible.
2. In season from as close to the source as possible.
3. As chemically and additive free as possible.
4. In bulk and not pre-packed.

Food Groups for Nutritional Balance

Grains, together with a pulse and/or nuts, make up complementary vegetable proteins. These include fats, vitamins and minerals. Herbs and spices added to these dishes stimulate enzymes, important for digestion. Vegetables dishes and salads, both cooked and raw, provide a varied range of starches, vitamins and minerals. Herbs and spices added to these increase the flavour and stimulate the digestive enzyme function. Condiments like yoghurt, chutneys, etc. are used to balance and complement other dishes in taste, nutrition, variation and appearance. The effects of improper eating manifest themselves in unwanted appearance, incorrect thought, behaviour and action.

In yoga, foods have been classified as rajasic, sattvic and tamasic.

1. **Rajasic Foods**: These foods are the food of a king, or of a restless and energetic disposition. A large

variety of foods having different methods of preparation such as fried, highly seasoned or baked form this category. Alcoholic and processed beverages as well as sweets come in here. These foods impart extra weight and fat to the body, and create a feeling of uneasiness after eating.

2. **Tamasic Foods**: These foods cause a lethargic disposition. Foods, vegetarian or non-vegetarian, that are prepared with excess spices, salts and hot seasonings are tamasic foods. These foods are characterised by a rough and intolerant temperament.
3. **Sattvic Foods**: These are foods which are cooked with minimum amount of spices or seasonings, and are fresh. These foods retain their nutritive value as they are cooked in a very simple fashion. One of the most powerful and delicious foods which has tremendous benefit on the overall system is sprout. Yoga recommends such foods.

Non-vegetarian food is tamasic, while vegetarian food is sattvic—this is a myth. No food by itself is rajasic, tamasic or sattvic. It is the preparation which makes it so. Vegetables such as cabbage, potatoes, etc., if cooked with a lot of spices, become tamasic, while fresh boiled chicken cooked in a simple fashion becomes sattvic.

Good raw foods, such as cucumbers, relishes, carrots, tomatoes, capsicum, parsley, together with spices like ginger, green chilies, cinnamon and basil, flushes both the mind and the body with pranic energy. Traditionally, raw foods, grains and dairy products are used for cleansing the nadis or the channels of the subtle body, because they bring with them an increase in prana. A combination of yogasanas, pranayama, mantra chanting, meditation and a yogic diet works wonders for those intent on cleansing both the physical and the subtle body.

Legends have it that the great yogis of yore live on air and prana alone! But it is possible for slightly lesser mortals to live on water, a little fruit and milk, and clarified butter (ghee) too.

Foods to Eat

1. Fresh, sweet fruits of all types, preferably taken whole.
2. All vegetables, except onions and garlic.
3. Whole grains, such as rice, wheat and nuts.
4. Ideally beans.
5. Not overly roasted nuts and seeds such as almonds, coconuts, walnuts, peanuts and sesame.
6. Butter, ghee and all good natural plant-based oils like sesame, olive oil and sunflower—in moderation.
7. Dairy products like milk, ghee, curds and cottage cheese from dairy animals that have been treated well.
8. Natural sugars such as jaggery, honey, maple syrup and molasses.
9. Ginger, cinnamon, cardamom, fennel, cumin, coriander, turmeric, mint, basil, fenugreek and other such sweet spices.
10. Herbal teas, natural water and fruit juices, particularly of the lemony kind.

Foods to Avoid

1. Meat, fish and eggs.
2. Artificial, processed and junk foods.
3. Canned food.
4. Animal fats, margarine and poor quality oils.
5. Garlic, onions and over-spiced food.
6. Fried food.
7. White sugar and white flour.
8. Artificial sweeteners.
9. Old, stale, over and reheated food.
10. Alcohol, tobacco and all other stimulants.
11. Artificial beverages and aerated drinks.
12. Microwaved and irradiated food.
13. Genetically engineered food.

Yoga diet is a perfect complement of yoga exercise. Eating properly will not only help you become healthy but also help you feel fitter and cleaner. Yoga diet also helps you regulate your weight, that is, lose excess weight and maintain a fitter body since it illuminates junk foods from your food list and includes only the healthy ones.

Yoga diet is a pure or sattvic diet. It is based on fresh and natural foods to keep the body lean and supple and the mind clear and sharp which is suitable for the practice of yoga and necessary in everyday life. It also helps prevent health issues like *diabetes* and obesity. Even if you do not intend to become vegetarian, we fully recommend everyone to follow the basic diet rules at it will make them feel better and be healthier.

Fasting

As a means of self-purification and self-discipline, fasting stretches way back in time. In nature cure, one of the very important tools for health and disease cure is fasting.

Many people are learning the trick of curing their colds, headaches, nervous spells and other acute troubles by missing a few meals or taking a short fast. It is the simplest and the most efficient way of relieving the overloaded and 'food poisoned' system. You would be surprised to know how little food is actually required to keep the individual healthy.

Yoga advocates occasional fasting, especially when you fall ill. In doing so, you give your digestive system a rest. You can observe nature's own precaution of fasting in the animal kingdom. Animals stop and rest when they fall ill. They rest and fast until their body naturally repairs itself and they are well again. Fasting on raw fruits and vegetable juices, from a few days to two weeks, is a common yogic remedy for many ailments.

One of the commonest complaints is that they have 'lost their appetite'. In fact, the greatest blessing to them would be to lose their appetite long enough to find their hunger. Loss of appetite is an indication that the system is overcharged with toxins and nature is trying to correct this by giving a chance to the waste accumulation in the organs to escape from the system. Fasting as a remedy is fully in harmony with the nature-cure philosophy of the cause of disease. If the disease is created by an abnormal accumulation of toxins in the body, it stands to reason that fasting will help in the elimination of toxins from the system. The membranous linings of the stomach and intestine which act as a 'sponge' to absorb food materials is now 'squeezed' to throw out the waste matter from the system. When you begin to fast, you may feel very uncomfortable or even ill during the first few days. This is because of the many toxins which are being released into your system, but soon after this phase, your energy and vitality will return.

Conclusion

If you follow the yoga diet faithfully you will find that you are now at a point where your sensitivity is heightened to all things that are occurring in your organism. You will become very aware that what you are eating has pronounced effect on the way you feel and act.

After some meals you will observe that you are alive and energised whereas others will leave you heavy, dull, lethargic in both body and mind. This is an important revelation. It will become very clear that the difference between the two states can be attributed to the foods you have consumed, and you will begin to think about eating not simply to satisfy your taste buds or fill your stomach, but for life-force. One grows more and more sensitive to the fact that light high-quality foods can give great reserves of life-force, help regenerate the body and impart many of the qualities of youth, while heavy, rich or devitalised foods can sap the life-force and add to the symptoms of ageing.

❑❑❑

14

YOGA FOR ALL

Yoga today is acclaimed worldwide as a natural way to rebust health, and overall physical and mental well-being. An interesting aspect of the practice of yogasana is that you get the thrill of gymnastics but without its harmful effects.

YOGA FOR MEN

Each one of us experiences stress almost every day, and men are not spared from this reality. They too experience stressful events from work or school, finances, family issues, and a lot of other matters, sometimes including the pressure to look good.

Men nowadays also experience the burden that they had been batting with over the centuries. Not only do they need to adapt from stress of being the head of the family or what others consider as the 'stronger sex', they also have to deal with the demand to look good.

Men are expected to be physically and mentally strong and fit to cope with stress and to meet the demands of everyday life, together with sports activities. To achieve a fitter body, they often go to the gym for exercises like weight training. A number of men also attend yoga classes to achieve a healthier body and mind, and help to meet life's increasing demands.

Weight training can help you in increasing your muscle size, strength, energy, and improve your posture. In the performance of some simple repetitive movements, you are able to focus work on a particular muscle or muscle group. These exercises initially damage the muscles which actually repair themselves and become stronger. Other benefits of weight training include decreased blood pressure, less risk for osteoporosis, increased athletic performance, and improved balance and coordination. The practice of weight training exercises combined with yoga can produce an even better result.

Given below is the basic yoga routine for men that can go with weight training, to help you obtain a healthier, more flexible body and reproductive system.

1. **Standing Side Stretch**: Benefits the stomach, the arms and the legs. Stretches the muscles.

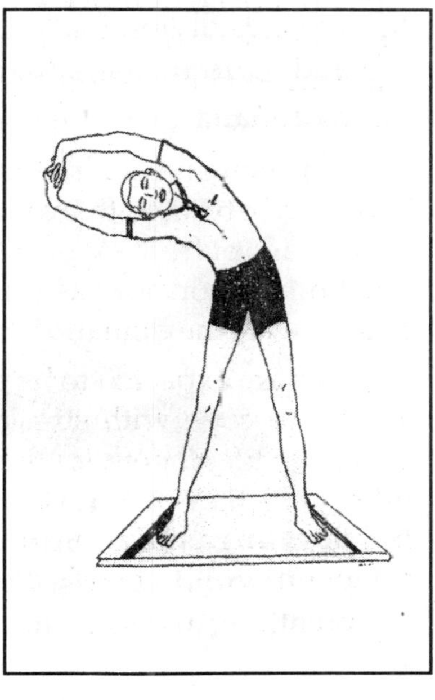

2. **Trikonasana (Triangle Pose)**: Laterally stretches the spine, tones spinal nerves helps in the proper functioning of the digestive system.
3. **Veerasana (Warrior Pose)**: Trims the waist, restores elasticity of spine, stretches the ligaments, the legs and the hamstrings.

Aids in the circulation of blood towards the brain.

4. **Ardha Matsyendrasana (Simple Twist)**: This pose literally twists and tones the spinal nerves, the ligaments, tones your abdominal muscles, and refreshes your lungs.
5. **Padahastasna**: Invigorates the internal organs, reduces fat, and stimulates the nervous system.
6. **Ardha Chakrasana**: Stretches the hamstrings and adductor muscles. Energises and calms your body and mind.
7. **Matsyasana (Fish Pose)**: Exercises the chest, tones the nerves of the neck and back, benefits the thyroid and parathyroid glands. Aids deep breathing and increasing lung capacity.
8. **Dhanurasana (Bow Pose)**: Maintains elasticity of the spine, improves your posture, increases vitality, reduces abdominal fats, and keeps the digestive and reproductive system healthy.
9. **Padottanasana**: Stretches and tones all the muscles.

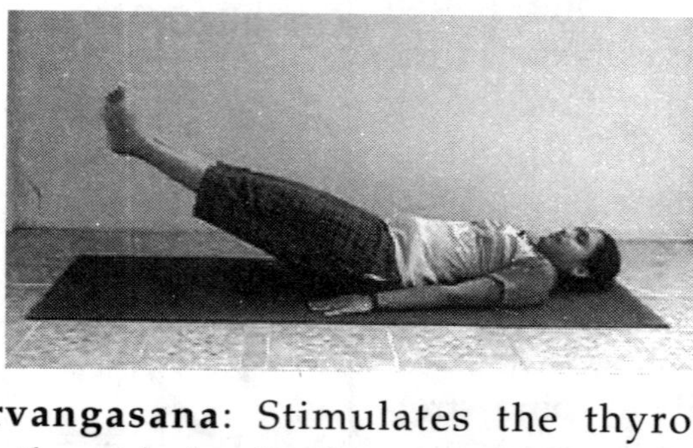

10. **Sarvangasana**: Stimulates the thyroid and parathyroid glands. Encourages deep abdominal breathing and stretches the neck and upper spine.

11. **Halasana (Plough Pose)**: Strengthens abdominal and lower back muscles, trims the waist and the thighs.
12. **Shavasana (Corpse Pose)**: This is the classic relaxation yoga pose that is exercised last.
13. **Ujjayi Breathing:** This strengthens the nervous and digestive systems, and gets rid of phglegm.

YOGA FOR WOMEN

Stress, hormonal changes and self-development are among the reasons why women should stay healthy. A woman's capability to handle stress, whether emotional or physical, highly depends on her health. The hormonal changes associated with menopause, pregnancy and menstruation can cause them to suffer from pre-menstrual syndrome, menstrual cramps, headaches and other symptoms. They also need to stay healthy to be able to cope with pregnancy and menopause, together with the symptoms. Women have also been under the pressure to look good over the centuries. Nowadays, a large number of women would do almost anything to be thinner.

Yoga, an ancient science, can help women cope with health issues and help them develop the state of their body and mind. It can help alleviate the pain that goes with menstruation, manage stress and ensure an easier delivery among other benefits. Yoga poses are also designed to tone and exercise the muscles of the body to eliminate excess fat, and make it more flexible and stronger.

Menopause is a part of every woman's life. It is the stage when your menstrual period permanently stops. This stage usually occurs between the ages of 40 and 60 associated with hormonal, physical and psychological changes. These changes can occur gradually or abruptly. it can start as early as the age of 30, and last until as late as the age of 60. It can also occur when the ovaries are removed or stopped functioning. Menopause is not an illness but a natural biological process, though the risk for heart disease and osteoporosis rises after menopause.

Symptoms include irregular menstruation, changes in sexual desire, hot flushes, vaginal dryness and urinary problems, changes in appearance, mood changes, sleep disturbances, palpitations and backaches. Not all women experience these symptoms. Some are not even aware of any other changes in their body. Estrogen and progesterone levels play the biggest part in menopause. In this stage the ovaries make less estrogen and progesterone. Estrogen is the female hormone that plays a major role in shaping your body and in preparing it for pregnancy, when the body prepares less of these hormones. The parts of the body that depend on estrogen to keep them healthy will react, and this often comes with discomfort in some women.

Menopause is divided into two stages: pre-menopause and post-menopause. Pre-menopause is the time when you begin to experience the signs and symptoms though you are still ovulating. You experience uneven rising and falling of your hormone level that often cause you to feel hot flushes and variations in your periods. Post menopausal stage is when you are about 12 months past your last period, and your ovaries no longer produce estrogen and progesterone nor release eggs.

Menopause does not really require medical treatment since it is a natural biological process. The menopause treatment actually focuses on relieving the symptoms of menopause, and in preventing any chronic condition that may occur during the menopausal years such as heart disease and osteoporosis. Some undergo hormonal replacement therapy (HRT) which provides a low dose of estrogen in the body which helps in alleviating symptoms such as hot flushes and vaginal dryness. HRT may also combine progestin with estrogen.

Women who have undergone hysterectomy only take estrogen replacement therapy (ERT) which is HRT using estrogen alone. HRT, however, has some serious side effects, and increases your risk to heart problems. Exercising, proper diet, not smoking and reduction of stress are also effective ways to make menopause more bearable, and can also facilitate in preventing any chronic elements that can occur in the post-menopausal years.

The following are the common health issues and changes that women undergo and the yoga poses that can help them through.

1. **Kapalabhati Breathing:** This breathing technique is specifically beneficial for cleansing. It can help cleanse the air passages to make you breathe easily.
2. **Parvatasana (Mountain Pose):** This promotes experience of stillness, strength, relaxation power and immovable stability.
3. **Padahastasana:** Trims the waist, restores elasticity of spine, and stretches the ligaments, the legs and the hamstrings. It also aids in the circulation of blood towards the brain.
4. **Veerabhadrasana (Warrior Pose):** Tones up the tendons and ligaments, the muscles of the calves, knees, thighs, hip joints, neck and shoulders. It improves blood circulation and the digestive system, removes headache and neck pain.

5. **Trikonasana (Triangle Pose):** Laterally stretches the spine, tones spinal nerves, helps in the proper functioning of the digestive system, and makes the body far lighter.
6. **Nitambasana (Side Bend Pose):** Benefits the stomach, the arms and the legs, and stretches the muscles.
7. **Rishiasana (Sage Pose):** Trims the waist, restores elasticity of spine, and stretches the ligaments, the legs and the hamstrings.

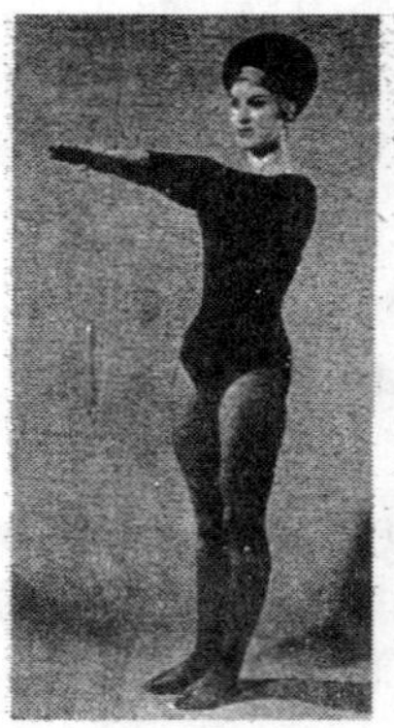
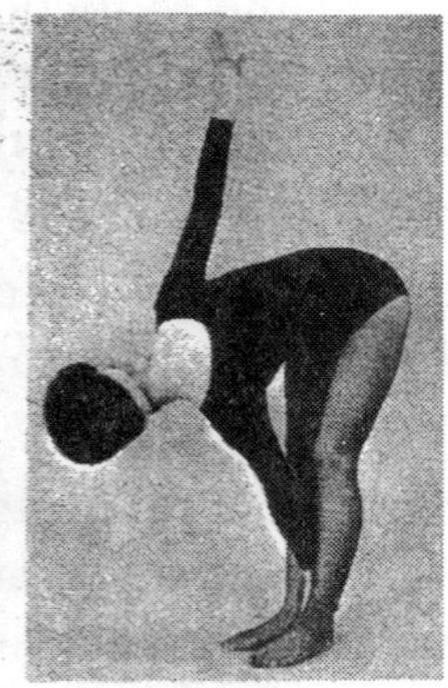

8. **Vrukhshasana (Tree Pose):** The spine gets stretched and limbered, and the muscles of the abdomen, arms, shoulders and chest are strengthened. It tones the nervous system and removes tension.
9. **Padmasana:** Excellent meditation pose to help you relax, to be more comfortable and alert.

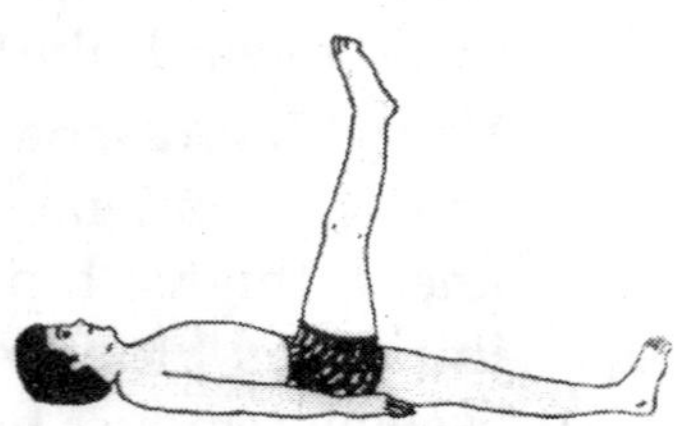

10. **Single Leg Raise:** Prepares the body for

asanas. It strengthens the abdominal and lower back muscles, trims the waist and the thighs.

11. **Double Leg Raise:** Strengthens abdominal and lower back muscles. Trims the waist and the thighs.

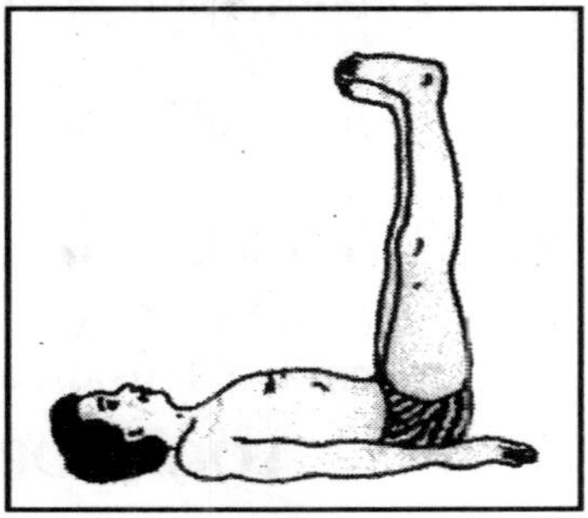

12. **Bhujangasana (Cobra Pose):** Coordinates movement and breath. Benefits the pelvis and spine, and stretches and strengthens the surrounding muscles. It also massages the abdominal organs, and is a good pose to combat menstrual irregularities and constipation.
13. **Ardha Chakrasana (Half Wheel):** Invigorates the internal organs, reduces fat and stimulates the nervous system.
14. **Naukasana (Boat Pose):** Helps to eliminate gas from the abdomen, and cures belching and hiccough. It strengthens the intestine, liver, gall bladder and colon. It is also good for women who are having menopause.
15. **Matsyasana (Fish Pose):** Exercises the chest, tones the nerves of the neck and back, benefits the thyroid and parathyroid glands. It aids deep breathing, and increases limb capacity.
16. **Shalabhasana (Locust Pose):** Helps in improving one's health, increases resistance and mental awareness.

17. **Sarvangasana (Shoulder Stand):** Stimulates the thyroid and parathyroid glands. It encourages deep abdominal breathing, and stretches the neck and upper spine.
18. **Dhanurasana (Bow Pose):** Maintains elasticity of spine, improves your posture, increases vitality, reduces abdominal fats, and keeps the digestive and reproductive system healthy.
19. **Shavasana (Corpse Pose):** Helps you keep more in touch with your body, and improve your ability to control tension and to relax.

YOGA FOR THE ELDERLY

Yoga is a form of exercise that adapts to your needs and abilities. It can be done even by elderly people and deals with your whole being, not only with your body but also with the mind and spirit. It makes your body fitter, the mind calmer and more relaxed. It relaxes the mind and keeps you more in touch with your body and yourself which can later develop to self-knowledge and lead to self-acceptance. It also helps you to have a positive attitude towards life.

Growing old is the stage when you have more time for yourself, your family, for leisure, recreation and relaxation. However, it is also the time when you are more susceptible to some ailments that are linked to old age, like arthritis, rheumatism, incontinence and high blood pressure. This raises the need for the older people to stay fit and healthy during this age, though the degeneration of the body also sets some limbs to the types of exercises they can do. This leads to the practice of milder forms of exercise such as jogging, brisk walking and yoga.

Yoga is also beneficial in the procreation and control of common health and emotional problems that are linked with old age. It helps you in keeping more in touch with yourself and your bodies, enabling you are in which creates a positive approach in life.

In practising yoga, know your body and respect its limits. Do not push yourself too hard in a pose. Yoga can only be effective if you practise it properly. The harder you try, the more you expose yourself to injury. Do not put more stress to your already stressed body. Remember that yoga aims to quiet the mind as you exercise the body. If you feel pain, stop what you are doing. You do not have to do all the poses, and remember to stop when you feel tired.

1. **Kapalabhati Breathing:** It helps in cleansing the air passages to make you breathe easily.
2. **Sukhasana (Easy Pose):** This pose straightens the spine, activates a sluggish metabolism, relaxes your body, and stills the mind, thus preparing your body for the different asanas.
3. **Adhomukha Svanasana (Dog Pose):** Reduces stiffness in the legs, shapes and strengthens the upper body, stretches the pelvis, legs, arms and feet. It also stimulates the nervous system, and rejuvenates the body.

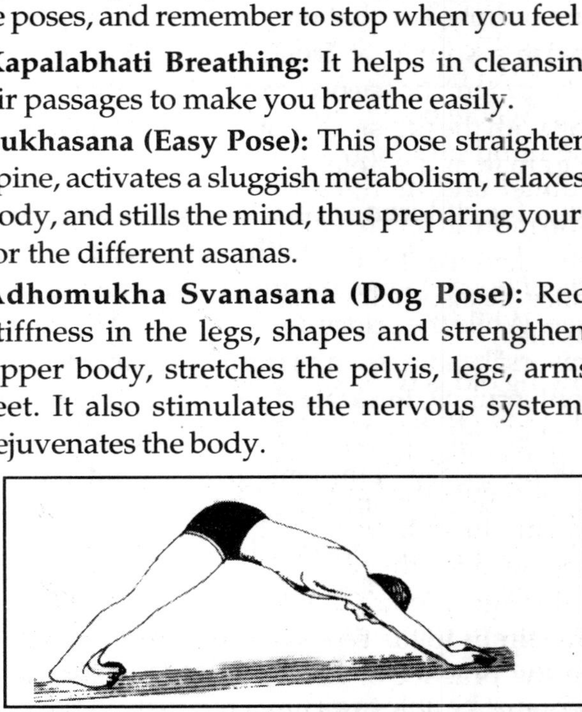

4. **Double Leg Raising:** Strengthens the abdominal

and lower back muscle. It helps to trim the waist and the thighs.

5. **Shalabhasana (Locust Pose):** Helps in improving ones health, increasing resistance and mental awareness.
6. **Shavasana:** This pose, after doing all other asanas, helps to relax all parts of the body, including the mind.

YOGA FOR CHILDREN

The practice of yoga includes a primary sense of measure and promotion. Each unfulfilled area of tissue and nerve, of brain or lung is a challenge to our will and integrity, or otherwise a source of frustration and death. Yoga is a timeless, pragmatic science evolved over thousands of years dealing with the physical, moral, mental and spiritual well-being of man as a whole.

Yoga for children is certainly one way to ensure that our children grow up healthy and happy of the many aspects of yoga. Yama, niyama and asana are relevant for children. While the principles of yama and niyama reinforce the universal values such as truth, non-violence, cleanliness and contentment, the asanas help a growing child develop physically, emotionally and psychologically. In this way yoga is necessary complement to formal education. By practising this wonderful science and art, children can blossom into healthy and well-balanced men and women with strong bodies, clear minds and pure hearts.

The role of the yoga teacher is of foremost importance if yoga is to be successfully introduced to children. The yoga teacher must be able to arouse anxiously in the pupils, and create in them a desire to learn. He or she must inspire and enthuse the children and should be cheerful in the class. A yoga teacher must, therefore, have physical agility and mental sharpness. The teacher should be a keen practitioner of yoga. Teachers and parents are often uncertain about the age at which children should commence yoga practice. Children aged eight years and above are fit to practise yoga.

Since children are supple and have no stiffness, they should be encouraged to do all the asanas for good health and agility.

Shirshasana (Head Stand Pose)

This posture is performed with the aid of a small pillow or cushion.

1. Seated on heels, interlace fingers.
2. Place hands firmly on pillow.
3. Place top of head on pillow. Cradle back of head and head in clasped hands, rest toes on floor.
4. Push toes against floor and raise body as illustrated.
5. Very slowly, inch forward with toes, and bring bent knees as close to chest as possible.
6. Place your complete weight on head and arms straighten back.
7. Push lightly against floor with toes; slowly bring body into vertical position.
8. In very slow motion and with complete control, straighten your legs, maintaining the balance of your body on head and arms.
9. Hold to 10 counts.
10. Come out of this posture slowly by reversing the movements.
11. Keep knees close to chest.
12. Lower legs slowly, with control. Do not come crashing down with feet banging against the floor.

13. Rest in head down position, knees on the floor, toes on the floor keep to a count of 20.
14. Relax.

Urvasana (Dancer's Pose)

1. Stand with heels together.
2. Place palms together on top of head. Elbows are parallel with sides.
3. In very slow motion bend knees and lower body, balancing the body on toes, heels raised from the floor.
4. Continue to lower into the squatting posture.
5. Without pause, begin to push up very slowly.
6. Straighten into upright position, remaining on toes.
7. Lower soles of feet to floor relax.

Kandharasana (Back Push-Up)

1. Lie on the floor knees together and bent, heels drawn.
2. Rest the palms on the floor, close to the head.
3. Push against floor with hands and feet.
4. Raise body a moderate distance.
5. Hold to a count of 5.
6. Raise the body higher as far as possible, keeping knees together.
7. Hold to 10 counts.
8. Slowly lower body to the floor.
9. Relax.

❑❑❑

15

Mental Health

What is Mental Health?

Mental health is far more marely the absence of illness. Mental health is peace of mind, and therefore, something we want for ourselves. When we speak of happiness, satisfaction, pleasant feeling, satisfactory adjustment to work and environment, economic, stability and good health. We are usually talking about mental health. Physical health is based upon mental health.

"Mental health is that state of well being in which, there is a dynamic, efficient functioning of the whole man which brings about co-ordination of his powers in such a way as to develop achieving his goals, both present and remote'.

—Dr. John R. Cavanagh

More Positive Approaches

Social psychologist Marrie Jahoda, who has made an exhaustive study of mental health, says that a person is mentally healthy to the degree that—

1. His attitudes towards himself are characterised by self acceptance, self esteem and accuracy of self perception.
2. He actualises his potentialities through personal growth.

3. His inner drives are focused and his personality integrated (the opposite of being fragmented by inner conflicts).
4. He has a dependable sense of inner identity and values, so that he is not overly dependent on the influence of others.
5. He is able to see reality—the world and other people with accuracy because his subjective needs do not distort his perceptions.
6. He is able to take what life offers him, he masters his environment and enjoys love, work and play.

Characteristics of Sound Mental Health

- The people who are mentally healthy, they are not bowled over by their own emotions—by their fears, anger, love, gealosy, guilt or worries.
- They take life's disappointments in their stride.
- They have a tolerant easy-going attitude towards themselves as well as others, and can laugh at themselves.
- They neither under estimate nor over estimate their abilities.
- They can accept their shortcomings.
- They have self respect.
- They feel they are able to deal with most situations that come their way.
- They get satisfaction from the simple, everyday pleasure.
- They are able to give love and to consider the interest of others.

- They have personal relationship that are satisfying and lasting.
- They expect to like and trust others, and they take it for granted that others will like and trust them.
- They do not push people around nor do they allow them-selves to be pushed around.
- They can feel they are part of a group.
- They feel a sense of responsibility to their neighbours and fellowmen.
- They accept responsibilities gladly.
- They plan ahead but do not fear the future.
- They welcome new experience and new ideas.
- They set realistic goals for themselves.
- They make their own decisions and do best efforts and get satisfaction.

Causes and Symptoms of Mental ill Health

The old Roman saying is, "A healthy mind in a healthy body". There are some factors of mental ill health—heredity, environment, physical and mental fatigue, distruction of cell tissue, psychological traps (drugs, tobacco and alcohol) and harmful habits, migraine, malnutrition, stress, anxiety, restlessness, ideas of inadequacy, inability to concentrations dwell on negativity self-defeating thoughts and psychosomatic conditions; lack of confidence and willpower.

Healing Needs

A person's mental health depends on the healthy satisfaction of love, care, understanding and affection, self esteem, belonging (approval, respect, and confidence), achievement (creativity, encouragement, aggression, determination and persistence), self control on anger, greed, hatred and intolerance, autonomy, (deep desire to learn new skills, dependency), Worship of God, atonement (expression of feelings, helping gracefully) (accept illness as a natural condition for human beings, encouragement do not argue, feeling of hope, rest and relaxation, take deep interest, helping positively (direct, indirect, retreat and evasion)

Change Your Attitude

From these negatives	To these positives
Fear	Courage
Failure	Achievement
Doubt	Optimism
Hesitation	Decision
Suppression	Fulfilment
Sour views	Enthusiasm
Defeat	Victory
Frustration	Gratification
Confusion	Clear thinking
Lonliness	Friendship
Inhibition	Daring
Scepticism	Faith
Cynicism	Hope

Discover yourself by doing a bit of honest self-probing

1. Do you recognise a purpose for your life?
2. Do you feel life is not giving you a fair deal?
3. Do you allow personal hate, envy, anger, and similar emotions to control your behaviour?

4. Do you indulge in illusion and day dreams?
5. Are you aware of your limitations of your capacities physical, intelligent and social?
6. Can you take disappointments and hard knoncks without being thrown out of stride?

Rules for a Sound Mental Health

1. **Maintain you physical health as well as possible.**
2. **Go easy on yourself:** Learn to profit from mistakes and failures.
3. **Don't expect to much from others:** Tact, curtesy, tolerance, friendship, good nature and sympathetic under-standing of another's personality these are the surest ways to successful social intercourse.
4. **Act with common sense:** Physical and mental health depends more on common sense.
5. **Keep youself rebounding:** Have cool head to maintain as emotional bounce to face a situation calmly and squarely, to meet a problem head on.
6. **Develop a social life adequate to your social needs:** Help others, love others.
7. **Keep Growing:** Carry on the harmonious develop of all your faculties. Within you lies the power to awake them.
8. **Man's greatest power lies in the power prayer:** "A Sincere prayer always is heared", says Sri Aurobindo.
9. **Develop your will power:** Will power is great inner force to do what you want. You can handle your problems due to will power.
10. **Self-determination and confidence:** Develop these

two powers. Once your confidence has gone your power has gone. Your achievement will never rise higher than your self faith.

11. Don't compare your self faith with others.
12. Be simple and contented.
13. Give respect rather than demand it, from others.
14. Control your passions.
15. Know that hardship is blessing in disguise.
16. Have only those desires which you can fulfill.
17. Deserve than desire.
18. Giveup sense of attachment.
19. Live and let live concede freedom of thought.
20. Read good books and have a good company.
21. Perform yogasanas, pranayama, mudras and meditation.

❑❑❑

16

The Art of Relaxation

Relaxation is an important skill. It is something that you do in order to rest, especially after work or effort. Everyone needs time for rest and relaxation.

The modern complexities of life with its stress and strain, hardwork and fatigue, conflict and tension, busylife and a constant struggle for existence, the common man many times feel tired and exhausted, constant activity need some sort of relaxation.

Relaxation is the most important goal of all the yogas and all techniques of yoga aim to produce tranquillity, posturers, breath control, mind-stilling mediation; the body, mental, and spiritual purification—all have a relaxing influence that is widely acknowledged as probably yoga's greatest advantage for the modern generation. Relaxation calms nerves, control over emotions and physical and mental peace.

Rest is the key of relaxation, quiet entertainment makes for real relaxation, too much activity and no activity—both are harmful. The basic problems are tension and hardwork, Relaxation, centre idea in modern yoga. Yogic asanas, yogic breathing methods, meditation, special psychological practices, yogendra Nispand Bhava, mudra and general relaxation are the sources of complete relaxation.

Basic Relaxation Position (Savasana)

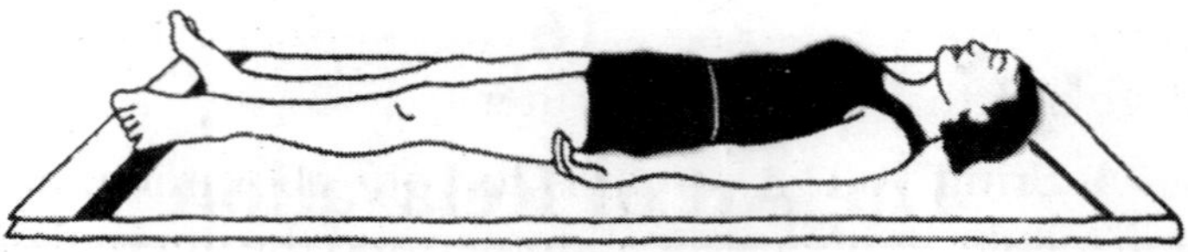

Method: The basic position for practising relaxation is lying down on your back. A warm soft blanket will improve your comfort and ability to relax to this position. Lie down with your knees bent and your feet flat on the floor, and gently press your lower back into the floor. It is important for your knees to be bent because it helps properly align your lower back. Put a pillow under your knees and thighs so you are not using your muscles to keep your knees bent. If you want to lie flat, begin with your knees bent and extend your legs one at a time without arching your back off the floor. Allow you legs to separate slightly. Place your arms down at your sides, slightly away from your body with your palms faceup. Pull your shoulders down toward your feet. Gently extend the curve of you neck so that your chin comes down slightly. Make sure your teeth are slightly parted, so that your jaw is relaxed. Close your eyes.

Relaxing Techniques

1. Begin taking some long deep breaths. After four or five breaths, bring your awareness down to your feet, curling your toes and flexing your feet. Hold this for three seconds and as you exhale, let go and relax your feet.

2. Now bring your awareness to your legs. As you inhale, squeeze and tighten your legs. Hold for three seconds as you exhale, release and relax your legs. Take a deep another deep breath and release.

3. Bring your awareness to your buttocks. As you inhale and tighten your buttocks. Hold this for three seconds as you exhale, release and relax your buttocks. Take another deep breath and release further.

4. Bring your awareness to your abdominal area. As you inhale, tighten your abdomen and the internal organs. Hold this for three seconds, as you exhale, release the abdominal area and allow the stomach to be soft and relaxed. Take another deep breath and release more deeply.

5. Now bring your awareness to your chest area. As you inhale, press your shoulder blades into the floor while lifting and tensing your chest. Hold this for three seconds; as you exhale, release your shoulder blades and relax your chest.

6. Bring your awareness to your shoulders. As you inhale, gently press your shoulder blades down in the floor, opening the chest. Then think of gently pulling your shoulders down, away from your earns and toward your feet, take a deep breath and release.

7. Next bring your awareness to your arms and hands as you inhale, tighten your arms and squeeze your hands into fists. Hold this for three seconds. Exhale, release the arms, relax the hands; and allow them to lie with palms up like gloves lying on a table, empty and still.

8. Bring your awareness to your face. As you inhale, tighten your face, crinkle your forehead, clench your teeth—make a prune face. Hold this for three seconds. As you exhale, relax your face. Release your jaw, and enjoy the tingling sensation of all the tension leaving your face continue taking deep long breaths, focusing on your exhalation and allowing your body to relax more and more.

2. Crocodile Relaxation

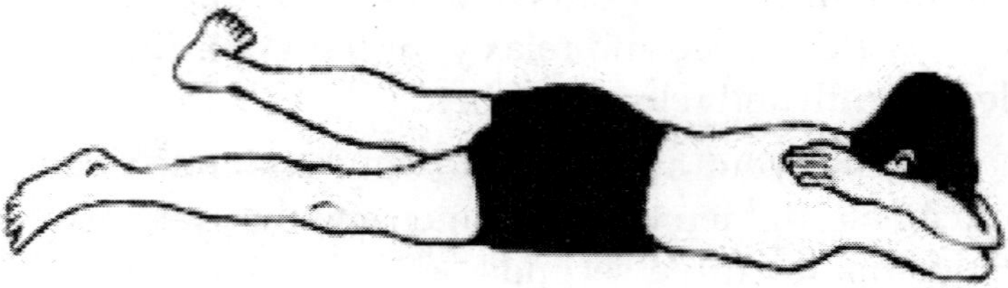

Method: Lie on the stomach, placing the legs a confortable distance apart and pointing the toes in or out, which ever is more comfortable. Fold the arms infront of the body resting the hands on the biceps. Position the arms so that the chest does not touch the floor, as pictured. Then place the forehead on the forearms. While inhaling feel the abdominal muscles gently press organist the floor; while exhaling, feel the abdomen contract. Let the body relax completely.

The Boat Pose

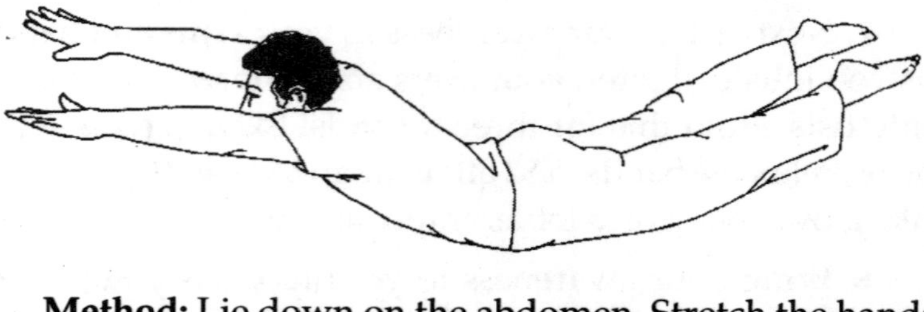

Method: Lie down on the abdomen. Stretch the hands beyond the head, inhaling, raise the legs, keeping the heels and toes together at the back and raise the hands in the front. Balance the body at the navel. Now start rolling forward and backward. During the entire process of the asana the feet and arms should remain fully stretched. While exhaling return to the original position.

Shithilasana

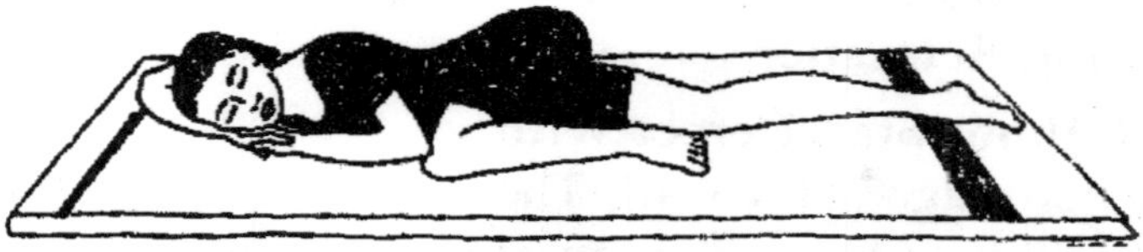

Method: Lie flat on the abdominal at full length. Resting the right ear on the ground. Fold the left foot at 90°. Bring the left heel to the right knee. Left hand palm may be placed in front of the face, shoulders are relaxed. Normal breathing with closed eyes. Repeat the same process on the other side.

Child's Pose

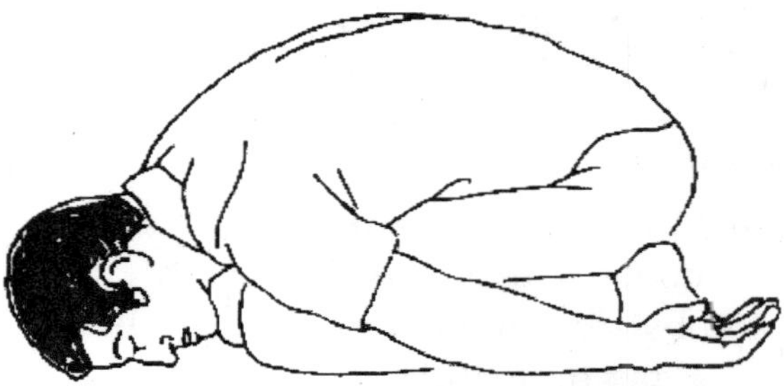

Method: The purpose of this asana is to adjust and correctly place the intestines in their abdominal seat.

Sit in the kneeling position with the top of the on the floor and the buttocks resting on the heels. Keep the heel neck and trunk straight. Relax the arms, and rest the hands on the floor with the palms upward and the fingers pointing behind you. Exhaling slowly bend forward from the hips until the stomach and chest rest on the thighs and the forehead touches the floor infront of the knees. As the body bends forward slide the hands back into a comfortable position. Inhale and come back stretching the hands.

Standing Relaxation

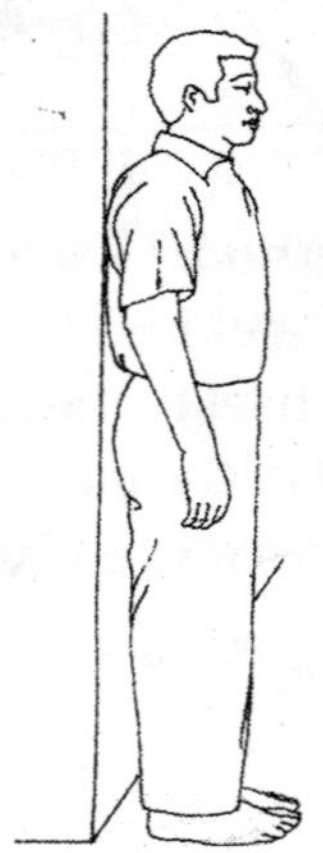

Method: Stand erect with your body against a wall. The heels will be a few inches apart from the wall and will be together. Allow the buttocks, shoulders, and head to rest against the wall without support, it is impossible to perform this practice to perfection. Relax the whole body head to toes. After reaching the toes, breathe slowly twice. Relax slowly and systematically from the toes to head.

Point Relaxation

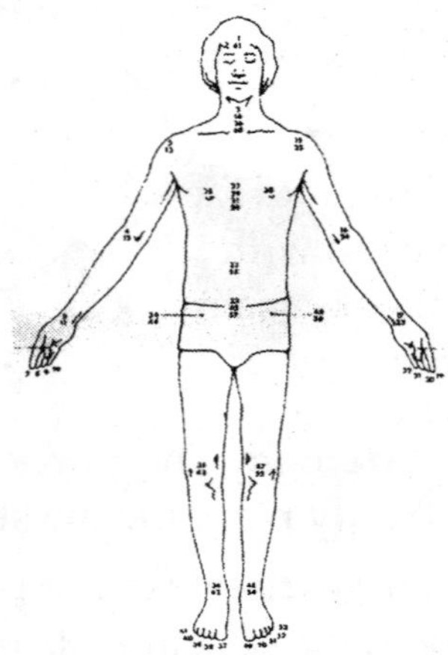

It is called 21 parts conscious relaxation technique. This includes 21 parts, step-by-step method to consciously localize different parts of the body and relax them in a rational sequence thus focusing the awareness in those parts. The different parts are—

1. Feet
2. Shines
3. Kneecaps
4. Thighs
5. Buttocks
6. Abdomen
7. Solar Plexes
8. Lower Back
9. Upper Chest
10. Upper Back
11. Hands
12. Fore arms

13. Upper arms	14. Shoulders	15. Throat
16. Back of neck	17. Back of head	18. Jaws
19. Face	20. Forehead	21. Bhrumadhya

Perform Jyoti Dharna and Jyoti Dhyana (concentration and meditation on the Divine light) at the Bhrumadhya Bindu (mid point between the eye brows) visualize the divine jyoti to be having the brilliance equal to 1000 suns but without glare. Absorb your self into this divine jyoti.

Note: Stay on each point for 3 seconds and feel the part relaxes.

1. This method is performed in savasana pose.
2. It should be performed for 10-15 minutes.

Advasana

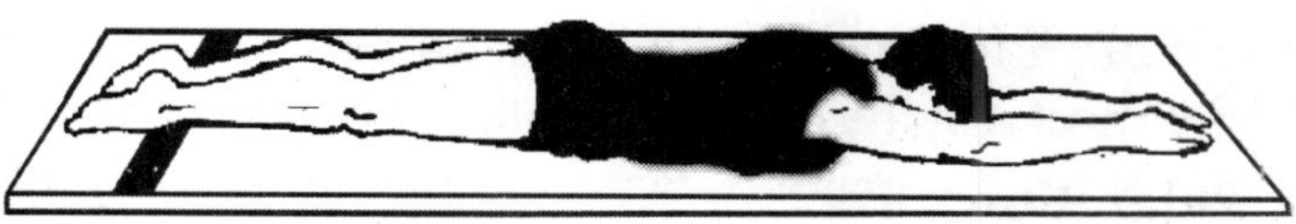

Method: Lie on the stomach. Bring both the arms above the head with the palms facing the ground. The forehead should be resting on the floor. Relax the whole body in the same way described in 21 point relaxation. If there is difficulty in breathing or a sense of suffocation is experienced, a pillow may be placed under the chest. Concentrate on breathing (normal or rhythmic). Perform for a few minutes.

Jyestikasana

Method: Lie flat on the abdomen with the legs straight and the forehead resting on the floor. Interlock the fingers and place the palms on the back of the head or neck. Allow the albows to rest on the ground. Relax the whole body and become aware of the breathing process as described in savasana.

Makrasana on Belly

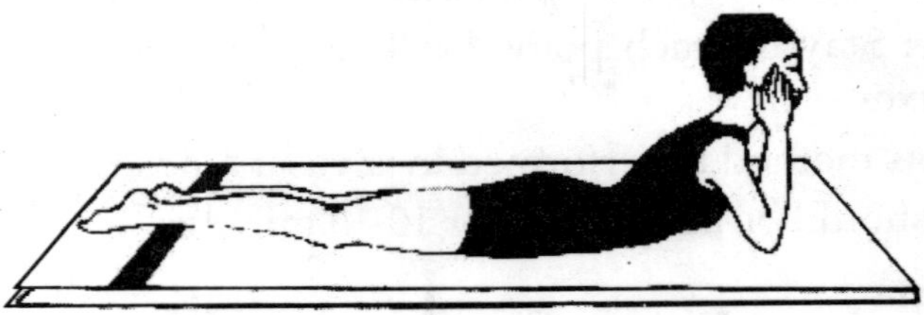

Method: Lie flat on stomach. Raise the head and shoulders and rest the chin in the palms of the hands with the elbows on the ground. Separate the elbows slightly. The ideal position is when the whole spine is equally relaxed. Relax the whole body and close the eyes. Have natural breathing and rhyth-mic. Perform it as long as possible.

Hastpadasana

Method: Stand keeping the legs apart. While inhaling bring the arms above the head. While exhaling bend forward with head and arms hold the ankles or put the palms on earth breathing normal. Repeat 5 times.

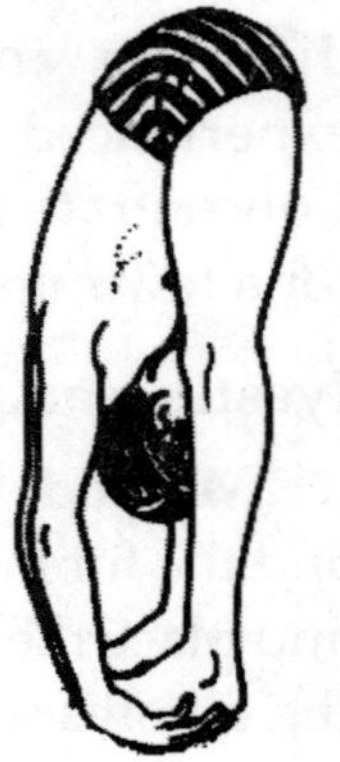

Note: Chakrasana, Ustrasana, Dhanurasana, Adhomu-kh Shvanasana, Setubandha Sarvangasana and Bharduaj-asana are also helpful.

Aswini Mudra

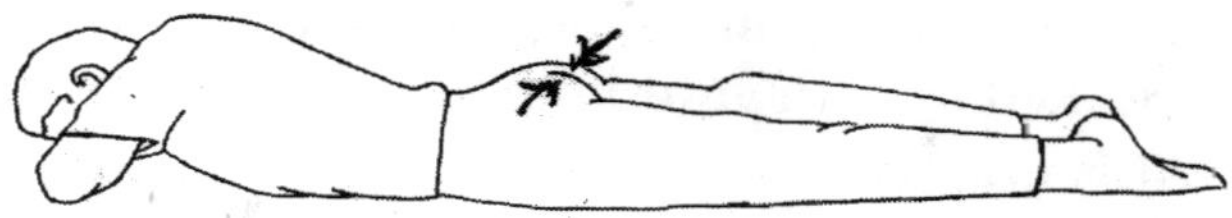

Method: Lie on the abdomen as crocodile pose. Bring the legs together. Slowly roll the buttocks inward. Increase the tension as if the anus in receding into the rectum. Tighten all the muscles inward, getting the effect of flattening the buttocks. The buttocks will be very firm. Hold briefly. Then slowly release the tension and relax. Repeat many times.

Agni Sara

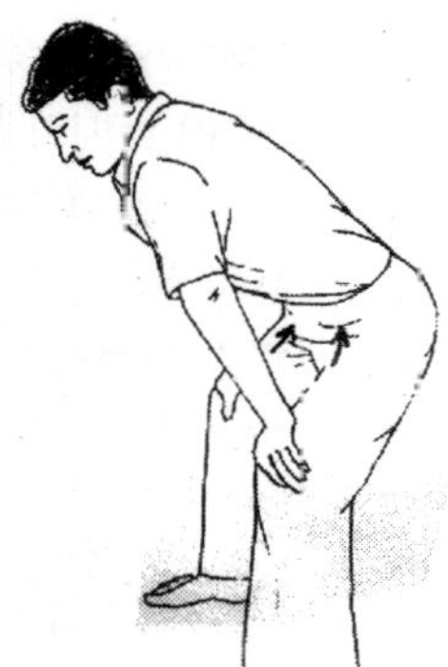

Method: The feet are comfortably apart, the knees bent, and the weight of the body rests on the arms. As you exhale, draw the pelvic area inward and up. Continue to contract this area as long as the exhalation continues. There is no retention of breath. As the inhalation begins, slowly release the contraction and let the pelvic muscles relax. Continue this systematic contraction and relaxation with each breath. If you tired or become short of breath, pause and breathe freely before continuing. Start with ten breaths, gradually increase to as many as fifty breaths or more.

Relaxation Breathing Techniques

1. Play some calm, soothing music in the background. Lie down for relaxation, close your eyes. Mentally scan your body for tension. Notice if your

neck, shoulders or back feel tense. Take your time. If you notice any tightness, don't judge it to be neglative. Just notice where you are feeling tense you checked in with your body in a loving way.

2. After you have scanned your entire body for tension, bring your awareness to your breathe. Imagine that you are able to breathe into each part of your body helping it to relax and open visualize the air you are breathing in traveling to each body part. Begin with your feet, helping them relax. As you exhale, all tension leaves your feet, inhale and visualize the air traveling to your legs. Your legs become warm and relaxed as you inhale. As you exhale, all tension leaves the legs. Work your ways up the body. Each time you inhale you breathe in relaxation. Each time you exhale, you release tension. Take as long as you want to each body part, breathing into the area and helping it to relax.
3. If you come to an area that feels particularly tight, keeping breathing into that area. Visualize the breath going straight to that area helping it to relax and open, with every exhalation, tensin leaves your body. As you work your way up, your entire body opens and widens. Your breathing is slow and even. You are relaxed.

Vigorous Breathing

Method: Perform child's pose. Take five deep vigorous breathing. The abdomen should be vigorously down in ward with the exhalation and fully expended with the inhalation. After completing five breaths, slowly come back to a sitting position on the heels. Let the circulation return to normal.

Ten Deep Relaxed Breaths

Lie in savasana. After completing 21 point exercise, have the feeling that your body is lying on the sands of a warm tropical beach. With the exhalation imagine that a wave passes downward through the body, carrying away wastes, fatigue, and all worries. With the inhalation a fresh wave passes upward through the whole body carrying a feeling of energy and well-being from an ocean of cosmic vitality. In this way breathe ten times. Then slowly open your eyes to the palms of your hands. Let your attention come outward to the space around you roll onto your side, and come back to a sitting posture.

Two to One Breathing

Method: Sit in any meditative pose or use a flat seated chair. Let your breathe become deep and diaphragmatic, and again briefly survey your body, releasing any remaining tension.

Make your exhalation twice as long as the inhalation. In the beginning count in your mind 6 or 8 for the exhalation while counting three or four for the inhalation. Gradually the breath will become more fine and subtle, and the count will lengthen to sixteen (exhalation) and eight (inhalation), or more. The numbers are given as illustration only, counting at about one count per second. Find the length of breath comfortable for you.

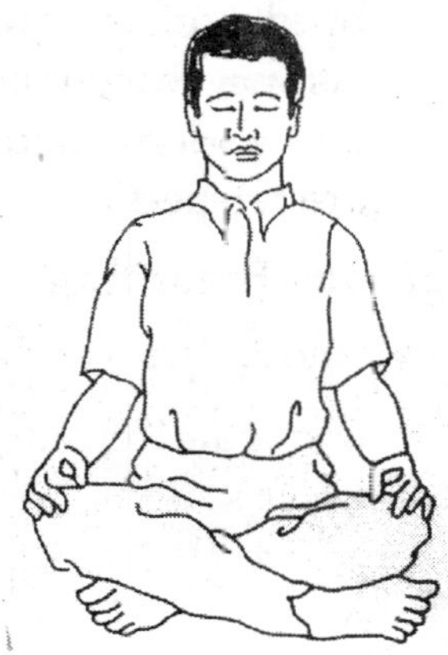

Begin with seven breaths, and increase gradually up to a period of three to five minutes. Experienced sadhaka may wish to continue with alternate nostril breathing (nadi shodhana) and meditation.

Note: Let the exercises become a part of your life and daily schedule you will enjoy all the benefits that the exercises provide.

Yogendra Nispand Bhava

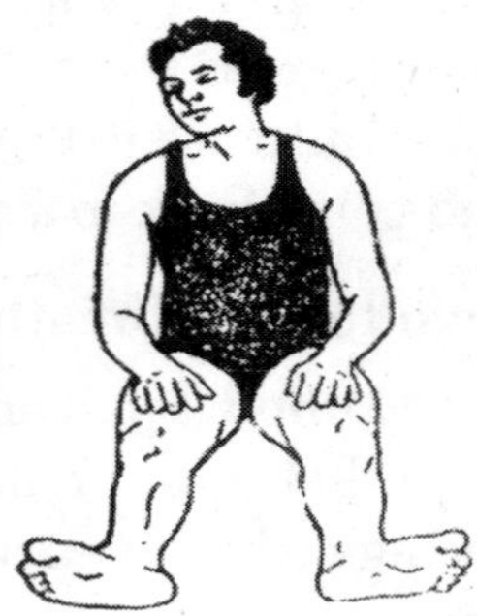

Method: Sit relaxed reclining against the wall. Properly adjust your legs, feet, arms and hands to a comfortable position. Sit motionless and feel quiet. Keep attention on sound—preferably a low intensity or fading sound or rhythmic sound for example of a time-piece. Cultivate the passive attitude of listening. Remain passive and get completely absorbed in the sound. Have normal breathing. Practice it for 10 to 15 minutes.

Loosing Muscles

Method: Lie down on the floor or one firm bed, loosen tight clothing. Support your head with a small cushion. Allow your legs and arms to lie loosely stretched out, arms next to your body. If you are suffer from lower back problems, put a thickly rolled up blanket under the back of your knees. Close your eyes and tense your feet and lower legs. Hold the tension to the slow count of five, and release the tension again, repeating in your mind the words, "Heavy and heavier sinking deeper" and, if you can imagine the muscles in your fect and calves relaxing into the floor or mattress.

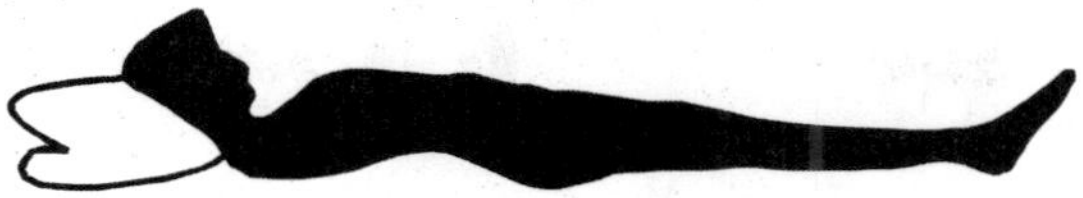

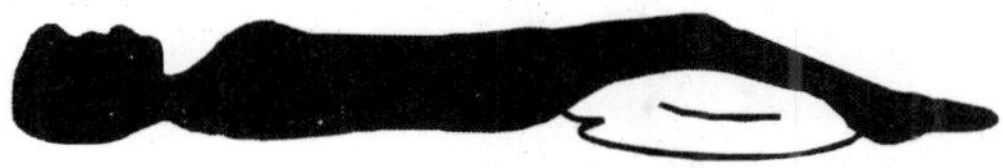

Take a deep breath in through your nose, hold it for a movement and then enable slowly through your mouth, making a HAAAA sound as you do so.

Give yourself a moment to feel the relaxation to your feet and lower legs. Now continue wih your thighs and buttocks. Tense them up tightly to the slow count of five then release the tension again thinking 'Heavy and heavier, sinking deeper' repeatedly as you let go, visualize the tension drifting away.

Take a deep breathe again, hold it and release it as before. Continue in the same manner for your belly area, your chest, hands, arms and shoulders together, and finally your face (grit your teeth and frown). This exercise has a highly relaxing effect, and this will help you sleep better.

Bhramari Pranayama

Method: Sit in any meditative pose. Keep the neck and spine straight. Close the eyes gently. Close both the ears with the thumbs. Put the first two fingers on the eyes, and the last two fingers on the lips. Inhale through the nostrils and fill the lungs with air. Now exhale slowly through the nostrils, producing he humming sound. Gradually increase the sounds. It relaxes the body and mind.

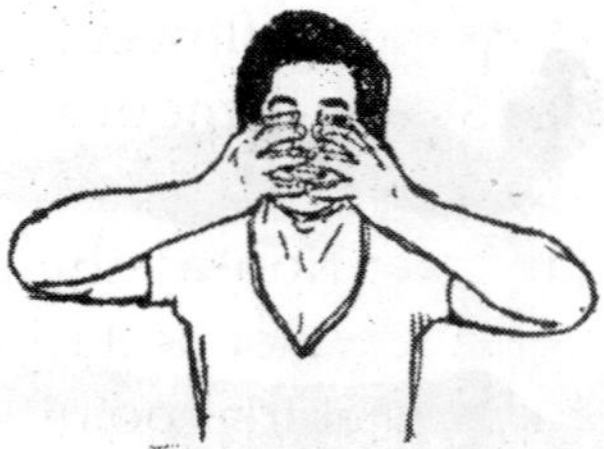

Relaxation of the Mind

Mental relaxation is the secret of physical relaxation. Unless the mind is relaxed, the body cannot be fully relaxed because the mind continues to function through the nerves, keeping the muscles and the organs of the body tense. One should learn the art of focusing the mind on the point on one thought.

Method: Sit in Padmasana or Siddhasana posture or sit in sukhasana or easy pose. Sit with upright spine. Older people can sit upright on a chair. Visualise he vast sky. Visualise the feathery clouds, the blue horizen, the sun in the day-time and the moon and stars at night. You can imagin any beautiful place, sweet memory and happiest day or event.

The following concentration exercises are used to achieve relaxation of the mind—

1. Trataka: The steady gazing without blinking at a picture of your deity or your ideal saint such as Lord Jesus, Lord Buddha, Shri Ram, Shree Krishna then close your eyes and visualize the form of the image from head to feet, and then in reverse from foot to head. Visualize every part of the picture in delail. Repeat this several times. Then fix the mind on any one aspect of the picture, the face or the fect.

2. Seated in Siddhasana pose or Sukhasana, with the

spine erect visualize a lotus flower blooming in the heart, in the lotus there is a steady flame of a mind without sorrow. Concentrate on it.

3. Focus your attention at the point between the eyebrows and visualize either nectarine moon or a radiant sun. Keep your focused at that point.

4. Repeat the name of the Lord or your favourite prayer to a malodious tune; then continues to repeat it mentally. Stop chanting and try to imagine that you are hearing the same melody repeatedly by arising from the depth of the heart.

5. Concentrate on positive qualities. When anger seems to overcome you, concentrate on love and forgiveness.

6. Writing the favorite Mantra in a copy as much as you keep the body in a easy pose. Visit the holymen, holyplace, study the holy book and meditate. These are also helpful activities for relaxation. Laughter theraphy is a good activitity for relaxation.

Relaxation of the Heart

Pray regularly. Feel the presence of the Lord with in. Be bathed in the grace of the Lord see the Lord in everything. Be detached from the world and be attached to god. God is the jewel of the heart, the soul of the soul the greatest friend, guide and teacher. Calmly surrender your ego at this feet and field his will. Relaxation of the heart requires a deeper life and a richer experience. Rise above the ego. Love all beings and be overwhelmed in bliss. When the heart relaxes, the soul communes with god.

Relaxational Exercises for Children

Here are four exercises inspired by yoga. Each exercise has a particular quality.

1. Concentration before the effort: It is a famous exercise used by countless, American business men.

Put elbows on the table, hands cupped in front of the eyes. Breathe in deeply and slowly breathe out. Repeat it twelve times evoke in the child a landscape or place the he likes. Let him imagine that he is there, one with the trees, mountains, sea or sky.

2. Attention and Imagination: Place an object in front of the child. Eyes should be motinless but without tension. Let him look at the object for 30 seconds. Then, with closed eyes, encourage him to see the object clearly. Then for a second time, let him look at the object in detail with open eyes.

3. Inner peace of mind: This exercise is based on listening to sounds. Lying or better sitting with the back straight and eyes closed. Ask the child to breathe six times, repeating mentally the word 'peace' or 'relaxation' at the end of each breathe. Then make him listen to the noises first in the distance, in the street, then in the house, in the room, but without trying to interpret them. A different way to practise for smaller children is to produce three different sounds, for example those of crumpled paper, a click of a ballpen and the sound of a step (when-someone walks). Then ask them in which order the sounds were produced.

4. Relaxation before sleeping: With the child lying down name the different parts of the body which he has to feel without moving. Start with the thumb of the right hand, move up the arm and then down the right side to the toes. Practise the same way for the left side of the body. Finish with the head. Then visualization of pleasant pictures to imagine.

❑❑❑